6-MINUTE
CORE
STRENGTH

6-MINUTE CORE STRENGTH

Simple Core Exercises to Improve Posture, Build Balance, and Relieve Back Pain

DR. JONATHAN SU, DPT

www.sixminutefitness.com

Contents

Free Bonus Material

I want to make sure you get as much value as possible from this book, so I've put together a few additional free bonus materials to help you, including:

- Videos demonstrating each exercise and their variations to increase or decrease the difficulty level

- Workout plans neatly laid out and provided in PDF and Excel formats

- A monthly email newsletter with tips to help you succeed on your health and fitness journey

To get instant access to all of this free bonus material, go here now:
www.sixminutefitness.com/corebonus

And if you have any questions or run into any difficulties, just shoot me an email at jonathan@sixminutefitness.com, and I'll do my best to help!

Introduction

You've probably heard about the importance of having good core muscle strength. Indeed, a growing body of science shows that core strength is essential for people of all ages and fitness levels, and that the real-world benefits of having a strong, stable core are endless.[1]

Having a strong core can:

- improve your balance and posture, keeping you standing strong and tall well into old age
- relieve back or knee pain and protect your joints from excessive wear and tear
- prevent exercise- or work-related injuries and make it easier to do daily tasks
- improve sports performance

In short, your core is essential for just about everything you do because your core is the foundation that allows you to sit, stand, twist, bend, lift, walk, run, and jump.

Clearly, you need to improve your core strength. So what if I could show you how to develop core strength faster than you ever thought possible? What if I gave you a science-based, field-tested approach that takes only six minutes a day — and what if you could see real results in just 15 days?

This book will show you the simple science of building core strength quickly, safely, and effectively with little or no equipment. No matter your age, weight, fitness level, or financial constraints, after reading this book, you will feel empowered to transform your body and your life.

Why I Can Help

I'm Dr. Jonathan Su, physical therapist, fitness expert, and author of the bestseller *6-Minute Fitness at 60+*.

Throughout my career, I've read thousands of pages of scientific literature and tried just about every type of treatment, technique, and exercise program you can imagine.

I've even coauthored the clinical textbook *Netter's Orthopaedic Clinical Examination*, which teaches healthcare professionals how to evaluate and treat physical dysfunction wherever it shows up in the body.

At this point, I can confidently say that while I don't know everything, I know what works and what doesn't.

What You Will Learn

- The muscles that make up your core and why they require a different training approach than traditional strength training

- Why an overreliance on sit-ups, crunches, and other forward-bending exercises may do more harm than good

- The importance of "core awareness" and "core bracing" during core exercises and most everyday movements, with simple steps to mastering both

- Over 25 of the most effective exercises you can do at home using little or no equipment, including variations to match any fitness level

- Workouts to address specific goals, such as improving posture, improving balance, relieving pain, and more

Imagine waking up every morning and feeling excited because you know your body is finally working with you, not against you. Imagine feeling more capable and confident in your body and ready to do all the things you want to do in life. All of this is within your reach, and it's easier than you think.

How to Use the Exercises and Workouts

I've designed the exercises and workouts in this book with a ton of flexibility and variation to fit the needs of just about anyone imaginable.

If you're new to core strengthening, getting back into exercising after a long break, or just feel like you need to brush up on foundational techniques of core strengthening, I suggest spending some time on part 2. This part of the book will help you understand and apply core awareness and core bracing, which are essential during core exercises and most everyday movements.

If you're experienced with core strengthening and you prefer the freedom of putting together your own workouts à la carte style, feel free to jump directly to part 3. This part of the book provides easy-to-follow instructions for over 25 exercises you can do at home using little or no equipment, with variations to match any fitness level.

If you prefer a more prescriptive approach to core strengthening, part 4 provides beginner, intermediate, and advanced level workouts that are a fantastic starting point for anyone wanting to jump into core strengthening without having to figure things out. These workouts can be completed in as little as six minutes. For those who want more exercise, 12-minute and 18-minute workouts are also available.

Part 4 also includes core workouts that address specific goals such as improving posture, relieving pain, building balance, and enhancing walking or running performance. If you don't find what you're looking for, email me at jonathan@sixminutefitness.com and I'll be happy to point you in the right direction.

My Promise to You

I've worked with thousands of people of all ages and fitness levels using the same program you're about to learn in this book. If you follow this program exactly as I laid it out, I promise you'll see real results in your body and your life in as little as 15 days.

Don't wait! Turn to the next page right now and begin your journey to the life-changing transformation that awaits.

PART 1

Understanding Core Strength

Part 1 will get you started on the right track by laying a strong foundation for understanding core strengthening. You will:

- understand why core strength is essential for just about anyone

- identify the important muscles that make up the core

- learn why core strengthening is different from regular strength training

- understand why performing too many sit-ups and crunches may do more harm than good

At the end of this part, we will discuss why short, six-minute core workouts are effective. I'm excited and humbled to be your guide on this journey!

1. Core Strength 101

I'm sure you have heard the phrase "strengthen your core," but what is the "core" and why do you need to strengthen it? Most people think of the core as simply the rectus abdominis muscles, otherwise known as the "six-pack" muscles on the front of the abdomen. But your core is much more than that.

The core is the center of your body, and it's made up of layers of muscles that surround the front, the sides, and the back of your torso. In addition to the torso, the core also includes muscles of your pelvis, hips, and shoulders.[2]

So why then do you need to strengthen these muscles specifically? Since the early 1980s, studies show that good core muscle strength is essential for just about every movement we do and activity we perform.[3] This is true for people of all ages and fitness levels in daily life and sports activities.

What Is Core Strength?

Core strength is the amount of force your core muscles can resist.

Because our society is prone to sitting most of the time, which results in potentially damaging levels of compression on our spine, we need a strong core to protect our spine from excessive forces that are present when we're sitting, standing, running, jumping, lifting, and performing just about any activity imaginable.[4]

When you stiffen or engage the core muscles, your torso becomes a rigid yet flexible cylinder, like a natural back brace or weightlifting belt, that offloads harmful compressive forces from your spine.

The natural brace created by your core muscles also protects your spine from potentially dangerous levels of bending and shearing stress from seemingly simple movements, such as pushing, pulling, bending, and lifting. Without the stability created by your core, the discs, ligaments, and bones of your spine can get injured and be in pain in the presence of these forces.

Additionally, the core is the kinetic link between your arms and your legs that allows effective whole-body movements.[5] Kinetic energy is the energy of motion, and your core is the link that transfers this energy from your arms to your legs and vice versa, allowing you to move in the world with greater power, efficiency, and ease.

For example, it would be difficult to sit up from a lying position without tightening your core muscles. Try to sit up without the use of your arms by bending your knees toward your chest and then kicking your legs forward without tightening your core. Notice how challenging, or even impossible, this task is.

Try doing this a second time while tightening your core and notice how you pop up into a sitting position with more ease. Engaging or tightening your core muscles makes this movement much easier because kinetic energy generated by your legs moves through your torso and effortlessly lifts your upper body like a teeter-totter.

In addition to linking your arms and legs, the core is also important for optimal performance during physical activities because all movements originate from your center and radiate outward. Golf swings, tennis serves, soccer kicks, and just about any motion that uses your arms or legs begins from your core and radiates outward to generate maximum force.

Why Core Strength Is Important

Because your core underpins everything you do, the real-world benefits of having a strong and stable core are numerous:

- **Helps you maintain good posture:** Most people with poor posture stand with their head forward, shoulders rounded, and torso slouched because of a weak core. By strengthening the core muscles around your torso and on the back of your body, you can then stand tall with your body in good alignment. The benefits of good posture are numerous, including reduced neck tension, improved confidence, and better breathing from having open airways.

- **Relieves pain:** Weak core muscles increase your risk of back pain and injuries. Core strength reduces acute and chronic back pain by improving support for your spine. Core strength can also relieve knee pain by keeping your legs in alignment when you're walking, running, or climbing stairs.

- **Improves balance and prevents falls:** The muscles in your core are key for helping you maintain your balance and lessening your risk of falling. A strong core helps stabilize your body so you can stay upright and reduce swaying that may throw you off balance.

- **Prevents injuries:** Your core gives you better control of your muscles, making it less likely that you'll overtax them. So activities such as carrying groceries, walking, running, and climbing stairs are easier to perform and you're less likely to suffer from injuries with a strong core. A strong core also promotes good body alignment during movement which can reduce wear and tear on your joints.

- **Boosts athletic performance:** A strong core is critical to sports performance because it enables you to maximize your power output and perform complex athletic movements with greater precision and control. For example, core exercises can keep a runner's legs from tiring quickly and allow a rower to pull harder and faster while paddling. The power of a tennis player's serve and a golfer's swing is from their cores more so than their arms.

As you can see, you need to have a good strong core. The good news is that building core strength is much easier than most people realize. In fact, that is the goal of this book: to show you exactly how you can reap all the benefits of having a strong core in as little as six minutes a day.

2. A Closer Look at the Core Muscles

It is important to get a general understanding of where the muscles are located and what they do. If the thought of anatomy or biomechanics feels intimidating, rest assured — you don't need to get buried in the details. I've included only the most important core muscles, and I describe them as succinctly as possible.

Some of you may still feel intimidated or overwhelmed by this information. Just take a deep breath and know that you don't have to memorize the name of these muscles, their location on the body, or exactly what they do. Just knowing that the core involves more muscles than most people realize will help you make sense of the exercises later.

Try approaching this chapter with curiosity, and I promise that this will make core strengthening a more skillful and enjoyable endeavor.

Movers and Stabilizers

The muscles of the body can be divided into movers and stabilizers. Most core muscles can work as both.

Movers, the big muscles on the surface of the body responsible for large movements, are the muscles that most people focus on when they go to the gym. They are the ones that let you do push-ups, pull-ups, and squats.

Stabilizers, on the other hand, typically involve much less movement and are the muscles that support your body. These muscles are usually much smaller and deeper inside your body than movers, yet they are essential for preventing pain, decreasing injury risk, and optimizing performance.

The core muscles are the main stabilizers of the body.

Major and Minor Core

We can also divide the muscles of the core into major and minor core muscles. The major core muscles are located at the midsection of the body, the ones we most often think of as being part of the core.

The minor core muscles are located farther away from the midsection. They connect the arms and legs to the midsection. While they are not traditionally thought of as being part of the core, they are important in helping the core work effectively.

Major Core Muscles

The seven major core muscles of the body can be described as a cylinder inside a box located around the abdomen, lower back, and pelvis.

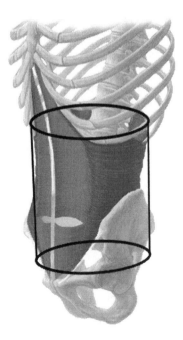 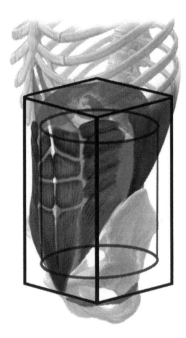

Bottom of Box

- **Pelvic floor:** Also known as the "Kegel muscles," this is a group of dome-shaped muscles located at the bottom of the pelvis. The pelvic floor lifts upward to help you control bowel and bladder movements and works with other stabilizers to support the spine.

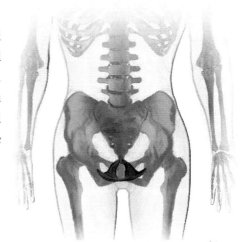

Top of Box

- **Diaphragm:** This thin, flat muscle sits under the lungs and is the main muscle used in breathing. The diaphragm moves downwards when you inhale and can support the torso from inside the body when you breathe all the way down to the lower abdomen.

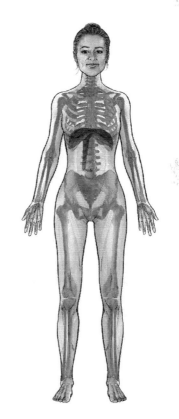

Back of Box

- **Paraspinals:** These large muscles on the surface of the body look like speed bumps running along either side of the spine. The paraspinals bend and twist your torso and are important postural muscles that help you stand upright.

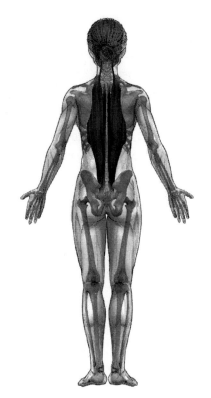

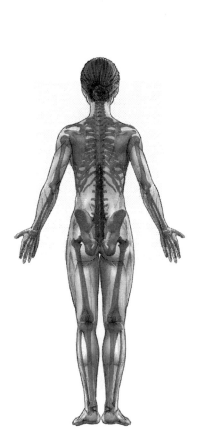

- **Lumbar multifidus:** These muscles also run along either side of the spine but are located deeper than the paraspinals. They are important for taking pressure off the spine. If this muscle is weak, you will most likely experience lower back pain.

Front of Box

- **Rectus abdominis:** This prominent abdominal muscle on the surface of the body is most well-known as the six-pack muscle. The rectus abdominis bends the torso forward by pulling the ribs and the pelvis together, and is an important muscle for posture.

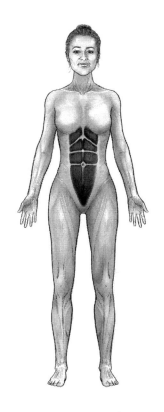

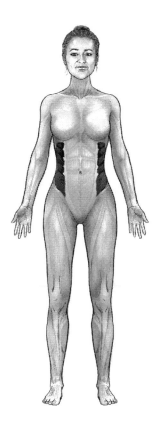

Sides of Box

- **Obliques:** These are actually two muscles, the internal and external obliques, located on the sides of the abdomen that bend and twist the torso. The internal obliques are directly under the external obliques and both work with other stabilizers to support the spine.

Cylinder

- **Transverse abdominis:** This muscle is the deepest muscle of the core and forms a cylinder inside the box. The transverse abdominis is an important stabilizer that works like a back brace or weightlifting belt to support the spine.

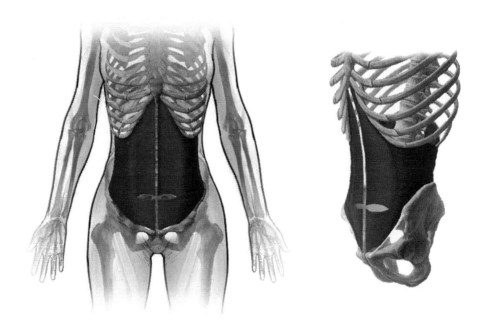

Minor Core Muscles

The six minor core muscles support the major core muscles during movements or activities. These muscles are located around the hips, back, and shoulders and connect the arms and legs to the torso.

Hips

- **Gluteus maximus:** These large buttocks muscles, located on the back of the hips, help you stand up from sitting or squatting. The gluteus maximus is also important for stair climbing, running, jumping, and maintaining an upright posture.

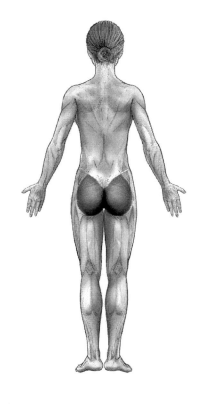

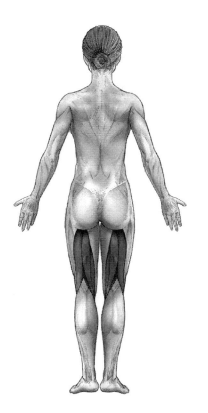

- **Hamstrings:** These muscles, located on the back of the thighs between the hips and the knees, bend your knees and move your legs backward. The hamstrings are important for pushing off during walking and running and for maintaining an upright posture.

- **Hip abductors:** These muscles, located on the outer hips, bring the legs out to the side. The hip abductors hold the pelvis level when standing on a single leg during walking or running, which is important for preventing knee pain and increasing performance.

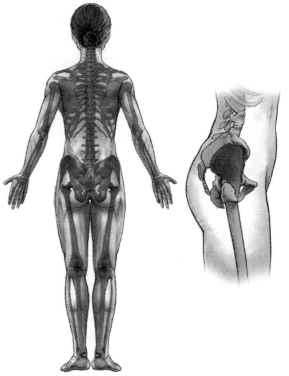

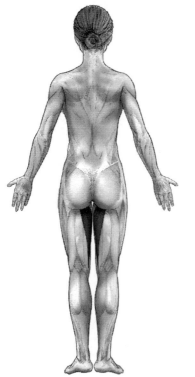

- **Hip adductors:** These muscles, located on the inner thighs, bring the legs toward the midline of the body, like the motion you make while making angels in the snow. The hip adductors are important stabilizers for the hips and pelvis.

Back and Shoulders

- **Latissimus dorsi:** This muscle connects the upper arms and shoulders to the torso. Known simply as the lats, they bring the arms backward and toward the sides of the body. These muscles are used during pull-ups and swimming and are important torso and shoulder stabilizers.

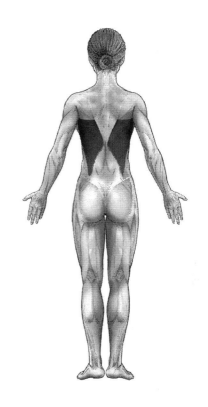

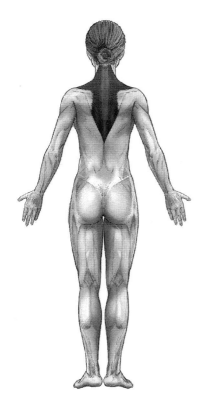

- **Trapezius:** These muscles connect the head and shoulders to the torso and work to tilt and turn the head as well as shrug the shoulders. The trapezius muscles are important stabilizers of the upper back and shoulder.

Remember, you don't have to memorize the name of these muscles, their location on the body, or even what they do. Simply knowing that the core includes different muscles with different functions is enough to appreciate the insights and exercises provided in the upcoming chapters.

3. How Training the Core Is Different

Training for core strength is different from training for regular strength because the former is focused on the stabilizers, while the latter is focused on the movers. The key difference between those two muscle types is this:

Stabilizers control motion, while movers create motion

Strengthening movers can be as simple as taking the muscles through a full range of motion against resistance until they get tired, while strengthening stabilizers is slightly more complicated and requires additional considerations.

How Stabilizers Control Motion

The core muscles are the main stabilizers of the body, and their most important job is to control motion in the torso, pelvis, hips, and shoulders. Controlling motion means preventing unwanted movements in the body. These unwanted movements are usually small and barely noticeable but can hinder performance and cause injury or pain over time if left unchecked.

Since our bodies are designed to move in a variety of ways, requiring our joints to have a lot of motion, unwanted movements can occur. So then the stabilizers activate and allow motion when it's needed and limit motion when it's not needed.

To illustrate how core muscles work as stabilizers, we can compare them to the lug nuts on the wheels of a car. Core muscles that aren't working as they should are like having loose lug nuts, which results in the wheels of the car being unstable. When a car with loose lug nuts is driven, the wheels will wobble, causing uncomfortable vibrations and poor gas mileage. Additionally, there'll be excess wear that'll damage the wheels and lugs pretty quickly.

This is similar to what happens in your body when your core is working less than ideally. There are three common reasons why it happens:

1. **The core muscles aren't firing (turning on) effectively during movement:** This is common and can happen because of past injuries, surgeries, or childbirth. It can also happen because of prolonged disuse of core muscles, chronic pain, or a lack of body awareness. Any of these things by themselves or in combination can cause the core muscles to fire ineffectively during movement.

2. **The core muscles aren't strong enough to control unwanted motion:** This happens when you lift or carry a load that is more than your core can handle. If there's weakness in one or more of your core muscles, it can even happen with simple body-weight activities like getting up from a chair or walking.

3. **The core muscles lack endurance for prolonged or repetitive activities:** This happens when you perform activities that are prolonged or repetitive such as household chores, endurance exercises, gardening, etc. Your core muscles are working fine at first, but they get tired quickly and are unable to work effectively.

Training the Core

To overcome the issues just mentioned so you can have a strong core that functions optimally, you need to train for core strength differently than for regular strength.

I mentioned how common it is for core muscles to fire ineffectively during movement. This is a "motor control" issue, and it's important to address it first and foremost so strengthening can be effective. (Part 2 teaches core awareness and core bracing to help you overcome this issue.)

Then once your motor control is no longer a problem, you can begin to develop strength and endurance. Muscular strength is the amount of force you can produce, while muscular endurance is the ability to produce force consistently and repetitively over a period of time. Both are needed for your core to work optimally, but the core requires a different training approach.

Instead of working against resistance through a full range of motion, like you would when strengthening movers, working through a partial range of motion or even no motion is the safest and most effective way to strengthen core stabilizers for most people. Holding a position against resistance without motion is known as an isometric contraction and is an important technique for core strengthening that's used frequently in this book.

Instead of working with lower repetitions using heavier resistance and relatively fast movements, like you would when strengthening movers, research shows that the core muscles respond better to higher repetitions using lighter resistance and slower movements.[6]

So you see, training for core strength is different from training for regular strength. So for this reason, the exercises in this book are performed differently than what you might be used to. If the information in this chapter is new for you, you do not need to memorize any of it because simple and straightforward instructions will be provided in parts 2 and 3 for you to skillfully perform the exercises.

4. Why Sit-Ups and Crunches May Be Bad

Sit-ups and crunches are popular exercises for working the abdominal muscles. They're the go-to for most people who want to strengthen their core or develop six-pack abs. However, sit-ups and crunches have come under increased scrutiny over the last several years. Many say they are potentially dangerous movements that should be avoided. But are these exercises really that bad? If so, what makes sit-ups and crunches so dangerous and what exercises should we be doing instead?

Too Much Bending Is Harmful

The idea that these exercises are dangerous is based on studies showing that repetitive bending of the trunk, like the motions used in sit-ups and crunches, damages the discs of the lower back.[7] These studies provide useful insights into how disc herniations (also called bulged, slipped, or ruptured discs) can happen.[8] But the findings of these studies should be interpreted with a bit of caution.[9] Why? Because they're all based on research using the dissected spine of dead pigs that were continuously taken into sit-up or crunch-like motions from 4,400 to more than 86,000 times using a machine in a laboratory setting. Based on these studies, well-meaning researchers began touting sit-ups and crunches as dangerous movements that most people should avoid.

I prefer a pragmatic approach when weighing in on these issues by considering both the research and the reality. We are, of course, living and breathing humans, not dead pig spines placed in bending machines for countless hours without pause. What we can take away from this line of research is that too much of the type of bending used in sit-ups and crunches does lead to damage to the spinal discs. But in reality, how many people do you know that actually perform anywhere near the number of sit-ups or crunches used in the studies? Some researchers may point out that it's the cumulative effect of these types of bending motions over a lifetime that causes problems.[10] In other words, there's a limit to the number of times you can bend the spine, and exceeding this limit ultimately leads to disc damage.

But we can make the argument that research also shows that exercises involving bending of the trunk bring nutrients to the spinal discs that are important for keeping them healthy.[11] There is a saying in orthopedics that motion is lotion for the joints, meaning the more you move your body, the more your joints are getting the natural lubricants they need to stay healthy and active. So these exercises can be beneficial. Many people have performed sit-ups and crunches for decades without any problems.

Who Should Avoid Sit-Ups and Crunches

Given that information, are the exercises okay? The answer to whether sit-ups and crunches should be avoided is more nuanced than a simple yes or no. Certain people should completely avoid these exercises. Others should hold off on them until after a stronger foundation of core strength has been developed using safer exercises. Still, others could perform sit-ups and crunches without short-term or long-term issues if they're done in moderation.

Who Should Completely Avoid Sit-Ups and Crunches

Based on the research showing that too much bending is harmful, certain groups of people should completely avoid sit-ups and crunches:

1. **People with back pain or a history of back pain:** Sit-ups and crunches are known to exacerbate back pain, and studies show a connection between back pain, disc herniation, and weakness in the core muscles of the back.[12]

2. **People with vulnerabilities of the spine:** Sit-ups and crunches can cause compression fractures in people with osteoporosis so should be avoided by anyone with this diagnosis. Also, those with more than a couple of immediate or extended family members with serious back issues requiring surgery may have a genetic vulnerability and should avoid these exercises.

3. **People who are older than 65:** Aging brings about changes to our bodies, often in ways we don't like. Case studies have reported strokes resulting from sit-ups, and older adults would be wise to avoid sit-ups and crunches.[13] Interestingly, research shows that you can find safer alternatives to high repetitions of sit-ups (see chapters 9–11) that are actually more effective at training for sit-ups than sit-ups themselves![14]

Who Should Hold Off until the Core Is Stronger

If you don't have any of the issues just mentioned, you don't have to completely avoid sit-ups and crunches. However, I do recommend holding off on these exercises if you're out of shape or haven't exercised in a while. After all, there's a connection between back pain and disc herniation, and weakness in the core muscles of the back. I've seen too many people who are excited to get back in shape who perform too much, too soon, and then are stricken with painful back injuries. My advice is to hold off on sit-ups and crunches for a few months and focus on developing a strong and balanced core using the workouts in chapter 14.

Who Can Safely Perform Sit-Ups and Crunches

You do not need to avoid sit-ups and crunches if you're in shape and you don't have any of the issues just mentioned. If you enjoy these exercises and want to do them, go for it! I would just like to make two suggestions, just so you don't end up in the group that should completely avoid these exercises down the road.

First, please perform sit-ups and crunches in moderation. Remember, the body has an incredible ability to repair itself but only if you give your body that opportunity. So avoid doing a hundred sit-ups and then a hundred crunches and then a hundred decline sit-ups and then a hundred twisting crunches every single day. You think I'm joking, but I bet I've just described some of your abdominal workouts. Instead, pick one or two exercises to do and then take a rest day away from these types of high-volume bending movements before going back to them again.

Second, do your best to develop a balanced core by working all sides of your core. Focusing too much on the abdominal muscles with sit-ups and crunches creates imbalances that lead to bad posture and back pain. Yes, an overemphasis on the abdominal muscles can lead to bad posture because it will overly shorten the muscles in the front of the body and cause the spine to round forward. This persistent rounding of the spine puts undue stress on the lower back, which results in back pain.

Overall, sit-ups and crunches aren't necessary for strengthening the core or developing six-pack abs because there are safer and more effective exercises, like the ones you'll learn in this book, that can get the job done.

5. Why Six-Minute Core Workouts Are Effective

Everyone has heard the old adage "Work smarter, not harder." In fitness terms, this can be more appropriately revised to "Work smarter, not longer." By working smarter, you can reap the benefits of exercise in as little as six minutes. Yes — six. Six minutes doesn't sound like enough time to make a difference, but studies have found that short bouts of exercise of six minutes or less, accumulated through the day, are no different than a single longer bout of exercise.[15] If the benefits of shorter bouts of exercise are similar to longer bouts, then why do I recommend the former over the latter?

Consistency

I like short bouts of exercise for one very important reason: consistency. The biggest challenge for most people in their fitness programs is staying consistent, and I get it. Most of us have busy lives, and we may feel too tired or unmotivated to exercise after having to juggle work, school, or family with all of our other obligations. However, if you want to reap the most benefits from exercise, you have to be consistent with it.

And it is easier to be consistent when you keep the workouts short. One study compared shorter bouts of exercise versus longer bouts of exercise in overweight people.[16] It showed that the group performing shorter bouts exercised on more days and for a greater total time than the group performing longer bouts. Not only that, cardiovascular fitness and weight loss improved more in the former than the latter. Clearly, shorter bouts of exercise will help you stay consistent with exercise and lead to better results.

After all, you can squeeze in shorter bouts of exercise throughout the day even if you're in a pinch for time. For example, you can exercise for six minutes in the morning and six minutes in the evening. Not only will this help you be more consistent with exercise, but you'll also likely see better results.

Supersets

You may be wondering how six minutes is possibly enough time to get a good core workout. It's actually pretty straightforward. We will be using a technique called supersets, which will not only save you time but it'll also make your workouts more effective.

Put simply, a superset is when you perform one exercise and then immediately switch to another exercise without taking a break for rest in between. Research shows that supersets lead to better fitness gains with shorter exercise times.[17] I love this idea because while I enjoy exercise, I also like to get it out of the way so I can enjoy the rest of my life.

With traditional strength training techniques, you typically rest for a minimum of 30 to 90 seconds between sets of an exercise (reminder: a set is the number of times a specific exercise is performed in a row). This gives you time to catch your breath and also allows your muscles to recover. But most people spend more time resting between sets than actually performing exercises during strength training workouts.

Supersets shorten our exercise time significantly by cutting out this rest break. It works because while your muscles are recovering from one set, you're performing another exercise for a different group of muscles rather than taking a break. You can switch back to the first exercise to perform another set and continue with this pattern until you need a break.

Cutting out the rest breaks not only shortens the duration of exercise, but studies show that it also increases the intensity of exercise.[18] This makes supersets a more effective way to exercise your muscles and cardiovascular system than traditional strength training techniques.

Core Strengthening with Supersets

Core strengthening with supersets is simple. Both studies mentioned earlier use a specific type of supersets called opposing muscle group supersets, which switch back and forth multiple times between different exercises that target different muscle groups on opposite sides of the body. For example, you perform an exercise for the front side of the core followed immediately by a different exercise for the back side of the core.

Another approach that technically is not a superset, but uses a similar principle, is called circuit training. It's almost exactly like opposing muscle group supersets, except you cycle through three or more different exercises targeting different muscle groups. For example, you perform an exercise for the front side of the core, followed immediately by an exercise for the back side of the core, then the right side, and then the left side.

The workouts in this book apply the techniques of supersets and circuit training for strengthening your core. That way, you'll get a more effective workout in a shorter amount of time — six minutes to be exact.

PART 2

Core Awareness and Core Bracing Made Simple

Part 2 introduces the concepts of core awareness and core bracing and explains why they are essential during core exercises and most everyday movements. This part of the book will also show you simple steps to quickly master core awareness and core bracing. Armed with this knowledge, you can then apply what you learned to core exercises and everyday movements.

If you haven't done so already, get the exercise videos and workout plans included in the free bonus resources by going to: www.sixminutefitness.com/corebonus

6. Why "Core Awareness" and "Core Bracing" Are Key

Core awareness is defined as the conscious awareness of your core muscles and is important because it allows for effective core bracing, which is the voluntary firing of the major core muscles — the muscles around the abdomen, lower back, and pelvis. Consciously firing these muscles during core exercises will make the exercises more effective and safer, protecting you from back injuries.

Developing good core awareness and core bracing is simple, but before we move into the techniques, you need to understand why they are important.

Movement Patterns

As adults, almost all movements we make are performed without much conscious effort. You typically don't have to think about coordinating the different parts of your body during daily activities because they happen automatically. For example, your opposite arm and leg naturally swing forward together while you're walking without you having to put any thought into it. This pattern of movement is useful because it makes walking easier and more energy efficient.

We learn several of these so-called primary movement patterns during the first few years of life. They include squatting, lunging, hip hinging, pushing, pulling, twisting, and walking. Primary movement patterns are foundational to all other movements the human body can perform and are refined through practice until they eventually become subconscious early in life. By making our repeated movements a subconscious task, we can focus on more important things in our immediate environment. Can you imagine trying to carry on a conversation with a friend if you had to consciously coordinate all the movements involved with walking?

Core Awareness Helps Dysfunctional Movement

While these movement patterns are automatic, they can easily become dysfunctional because of injury, disuse, or other changes to our bodies. For example, an injury such as a sprained ankle will force us to alter our movement patterns to compensate for the pain. Prolonged disuse from sitting at a desk at work or on a couch in front of a TV for hours every day can cause the brain to simply forget how our body was meant to move. Changes to our body because of pregnancy or weight gain can also leave lasting effects on our movement patterns that are not ideal.

Most people don't realize that dysfunctional movement patterns can stay with us even after injury, disuse, or other changes to our bodies unless we make a conscious effort to correct them. It's no wonder poor posture, aches and pains, joint wear and tear, and suboptimal physical performance seem to creep up on us over time as we experience seemingly insignificant injuries, periods of disuse, and other changes.

The good news is that you can easily correct dysfunctional movement patterns through motor learning, and the key ingredient is awareness. Motor learning is the process of learning new patterns of movement. When you bring your conscious awareness to movement that is slow and intentional, your brain switches into learning mode that allows new movement patterns to be programmed. This is a gradual process that requires more conscious effort at first but becomes automatic over time.

Core awareness is motor learning with the goal of teaching or reteaching the brain how to fire the core muscles. Research shows that the major core muscles are designed to automatically fire milliseconds before any voluntary movement of the body.[19] This provides your body the support it needs to make movements safe, efficient, and powerful. I find that most adults, no matter their fitness level, have some level of dysfunctional movement patterns of the core muscles that leaves the body vulnerable to pain, injuries, and poor performance. I'll show you six simple steps to develop core awareness in the next chapter.

Core Bracing and Motor Control

Firing the major core muscles of your abdomen, lower back, and pelvis during movement or activities should ideally be done automatically. But if the movement or activity is new, complex, or strenuous, the core muscles may not fire effectively. This can also happen with simple movements or familiar activities that happen unexpectedly. For example, it's common for people to tweak their backs with sudden movements like missing a step or bending over to pick up something while not paying attention to their movement.

In these situations, it's as if the brain is asleep at the wheel and forgets to fire the core muscles effectively. This is known as a motor control issue, and the solution is core bracing. Motor control is the ability to execute purposeful movement to carry out a goal. By firing these muscles on command, core bracing develops motor control of the core. This technique is used in sports and strength training all the time, and it'll protect your back during core exercises and make the exercises more effective. It'll also make everyday movements and activities safer and easier to perform. I'll show you how to master core bracing in a snap in chapter 8.

7. Six Steps to Developing Good Core Awareness

The six steps to developing good core awareness remind your brain how to fire your core muscles and how your body was meant to move:

1. Centering
2. Awareness of spine motion
3. Awareness of pelvic floor muscles
4. Awareness of abdominal muscles
5. Awareness of back muscles
6. Belly breathing

Step 1: Centering

Centering shifts your brain into a calm yet focused state, which will boost its ability to learn.

1. Find a quiet and comfortable spot with enough room to lie on your back with your arms and legs spread wide. A firm bed or an exercise mat on the floor would be ideal.

2. Close your eyes and take a moment to breathe a little deeper and a little slower than you normally would.

3. Bring your awareness to your body from head to toe and skin to bone. Notice any tension you might be holding and see if you can let it go.

Step 2: Awareness of Spine Motion

This step develops awareness of how the motion of the spine, pelvis, and shoulders are connected.

Pelvis Motion

Because the pelvis is connected directly to the lumbar (lower) spine, too much tilting in either direction can place stress on the lower back. Imagine the pelvis as a bucket filled with water that can tilt forward and backward. Water will spill if the bucket tilts too much in either direction. Practice the following steps to explore the connection between pelvis and spine motion.

1. Lie on your back with your knees bent and the soles of your feet on the floor slightly apart.

2. Place your hands next to your hips with your palms resting on the floor.

3. Gently rock your pelvis backward so your lower back presses into the floor. This backward tilting of the pelvis flattens the curve of your lower back.

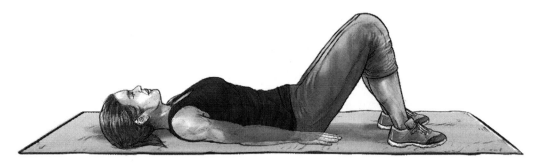

4. Gently rock your pelvis forward (in the opposite direction) so your lower back arches or lifts off the floor. This forward tilting of the pelvis exaggerates the curve in your lower back.

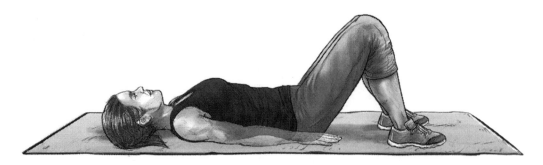

5. Repeat these motions slowly and intentionally three times while noticing which position between the two extremes of motion is most comfortable for your lower back. This position is your pelvic neutral.

Pelvic neutral is the most comfortable and safest position for your lower back. We'll be using these steps to "find pelvic neutral" in the next chapter.

Shoulder Motion

Because the shoulder is connected to your thoracic (upper) spine, too much forward motion causes your spine to round forward, which is common in people with poor posture. Too much backward motion causes your spine to arch backward, which can place stress on your lower back. Practice the following steps to explore the connection between your shoulder and spine motion.

1. Lie on your back with your knees bent and the soles of your feet on the floor slightly apart.

2. Place your hands next to your hips with your palms resting on the floor.

3. Lift your head off the floor and move your shoulders forward (toward the ceiling) and together. Notice how moving your shoulders forward also rounds your spine.

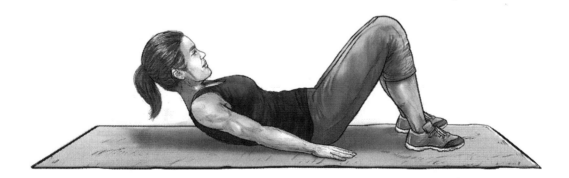

4. Return your head on the floor and move your shoulders backward (toward the floor) and together. Push your elbows against the floor to assist with this motion. Notice how moving your shoulders backward arches your spine.

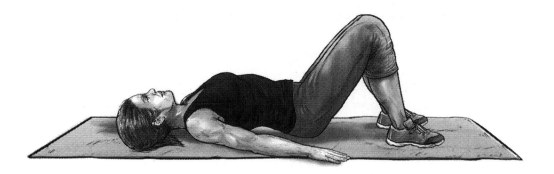

5. Repeat these motions slowly and intentionally three times while noticing which part of the motion is most comfortable for your spine.

A large part of good posture is ensuring that your shoulders are in a neutral position that's not too far forward or backward.

Step 3: Awareness of Pelvic Floor Muscles

The pelvic floor muscles at the bottom of your pelvis should fire during core bracing. Practice the following steps to remind your brain how to fire these muscles.

1. Lie on your back with your knees bent and the soles of your feet on the floor slightly apart. Bring your awareness to your pelvic floor area at the bottom of your pelvis.

2. Fire your pelvic floor muscles by imagining that you have to urinate and then stopping the flow of urine. Notice the muscles at the bottom of your pelvis tighten and lift when you do this.

3. Alternate between firing your pelvic floor muscles continuously for three seconds and relaxing them completely for three seconds. Repeat this five times and notice how it feels.

4. Fire your pelvic floor muscles continuously for 15 seconds and notice the sensations you feel. This is called "firing and holding" and is an important part of core bracing.

Step 4: Awareness of Abdominal Muscles

The abdominal muscles should also fire during core bracing. Practice the steps below to help feel what happens in your body when you fire these muscles.

1. Lie on your back with your knees bent and the soles of your feet on the floor slightly apart.

2. Place your fingers on either side of your belly button, about one inch away from the center.

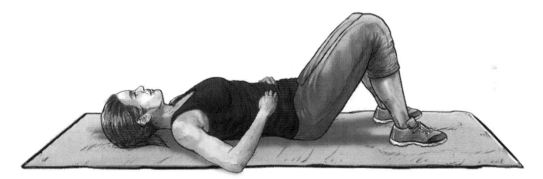

3. Fire your abdominal muscles as if you're bracing for a punch, and notice your abdominal muscles tighten under your fingers.

4. Alternate between firing your abdominal muscles continuously for three seconds and relaxing them completely for three seconds. Repeat this five times and notice how your abdominal muscles feel under your fingers.

5. Fire and hold your abdominal muscles for 15 seconds and notice how it feels.

Step 5: Awareness of Back Muscles

The lower back muscles should fire during core bracing. The easiest way to fire these muscles is to fire your abdominal muscles forcefully. While it may be more difficult to feel your lower back muscles fire, don't worry; you'll get better with practice.

1. Lie on your back with your knees bent and the soles of your feet on the floor slightly apart.

2. Place your fingers on your lower back muscles on either side of your spine, about one inch away from the center.

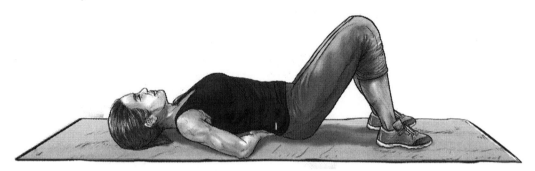

3. Fire your abdominal muscles forcefully as if you're bracing for a punch and see if you can notice your lower back muscles tighten under your fingers. You can try coughing a few times to get the muscles to engage more forcefully if you have trouble feeling the muscles firing.

4. Alternate between firing your abdominal muscles continuously for three seconds and relaxing your muscles completely for three seconds. Repeat this five times and notice how your lower back muscles feel under your fingers.

5. Fire and hold your abdominal muscles for 15 seconds and notice how your lower back muscles feel.

Step 6: Belly Breathing

Your diaphragm is the main muscle used for breathing, and it plays an important role during core bracing when belly breathing is used.

1. Lie on your back with your knees bent and the soles of your feet on the floor slightly apart.

2. Place the palm of one hand on your chest and the palm of the other hand on your belly button. Breathe as you normally would and notice that your chest moves more than your belly. This is called chest breathing, and it does not help stabilize your core.

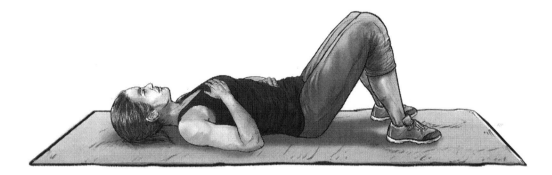

3. Breathe down to your belly button and feel your lower abdomen expand into your fingers as you inhale while your chest remains still. This is called belly breathing, and it helps stabilize the core by increasing the pressure inside your torso when you breathe.

4. Practice belly breathing by taking three seconds to inhale and three seconds to exhale while your lower abdomen expands and your chest remains still. Repeat five times.

I suggest spending about a minute on each step and completing all six steps in one sitting. Try practicing at least once daily for two or three days before moving to the next chapter. I encourage you to approach each step slowly and intentionally as if you were an explorer discovering something new. This will ensure that you'll bring the conscious awareness needed for your brain to switch into learning mode.

Don't worry if you feel like you're not "getting it" or if you feel like nothing is "happening." Process is more important than outcome when it comes to developing core awareness. In other words, you don't have to feel like you're getting it or that anything is happening because your brain will learn how to move and how to fire your core muscles by simply going through the steps with conscious awareness.

8. Core Bracing (the Right Way) from Beginner to Advanced

Core bracing is a simple technique that involves firing the muscles of your abdomen, lower back, and pelvis on command. Core bracing is effective for reducing pain, preventing injuries, and improving performance during core exercises and more strenuous movements in daily life. Some amount of core bracing is always unconsciously happening during any movement. But as we discussed in chapter 6, the brain sometimes forgets, or the body is unable to effectively brace because of a history of injury, disuse, or other changes to our bodies. By learning core bracing the right way, you'll do it with a conscious effort at first. Over time, you'll be able to effectively brace your core with little or no conscious effort.

There are two levels of core bracing techniques: beginner and advanced. Work through each level in sequence, and after completing this chapter, you'll be able to tackle core strengthening exercises safely and effectively and immediately use core bracing in your daily life to improve posture, relieve pain, and increase performance.

Try practicing for about six minutes at least once daily for two or three days on beginner core bracing. Do the same on advanced core bracing before moving to the next chapter. Practice two or three times a day if you have time. Remember to approach each step slowly and intentionally, as if you were an explorer discovering something new. This will ensure that you'll bring the conscious awareness needed for your brain to switch into learning mode.

Beginner Core Bracing

You'll recognize the steps here from the previous chapter on core awareness, so there's nothing new except for putting those pieces together.

1. Lie on your back with your knees bent and the soles of your feet on the floor slightly apart.

2. Place the fingers of your left and right hand on either side of your belly button, about one inch away from the center. Gently rock your pelvis backward and forward a few times to find pelvic neutral.

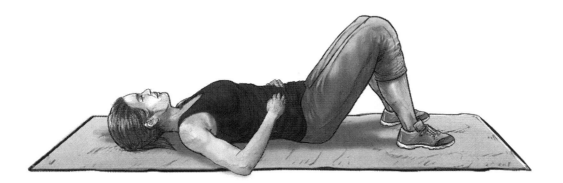

3. Fire your pelvic floor muscles by pretending that you have to urinate and then stopping the flow of urine. Notice the pelvic floor muscles tighten and lift when you do this.

4. While keeping your pelvic floor muscles firing, fire your abdominal muscles as if you're bracing for a punch and notice your abdominal muscles tighten under your fingers.

5. While keeping your pelvic floor and abdominal muscles firing, begin belly breathing by breathing all the way down to the belly button. Use your fingers to monitor the stiffness of your abdominal muscles to ensure you're maintaining an effective brace as you inhale and exhale five times at a normal pace.

6. Stop what you're doing, and completely relax for 30 seconds to allow your brain a chance to integrate this work. Repeat these steps three to five times.

Move to advanced core bracing once you have this level down, or after three days, even if you don't feel like you have it completely down.

Advanced Core Bracing

Adding arm and leg movements increases the challenge of core bracing because it forces the brain to focus on multiple things at one time. This type of challenge more closely resembles the challenges of core bracing in real life. Work in the sequence provided from leg movement, to arm movement, and ending with combined movement.

Leg Movement

1. Lie on your back with your knees bent and the soles of your feet on the floor slightly apart.

2. Place the fingers of your left and right hand on either side of your belly button, about one inch away from the center to feel your lower abdomen tighten when you brace. Gently rock your pelvis backward and forward a few times to find pelvic neutral.

3. Brace your core by lifting your pelvic floor, tightening your abdomen, and breathing to your belly button.

4. Slowly slide your right heel forward on the floor until your leg is straight, and then slide it back to the starting position. Repeat this same motion with your left leg.

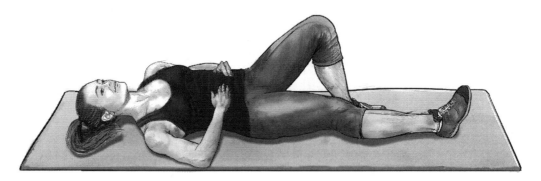

5. Slowly bring your right knee toward your chest, and then bring it back to the starting position. Repeat this same motion with your left leg.

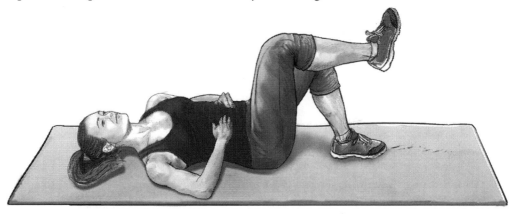

6. Repeat these motions three times while ensuring your pelvis and torso remain still and your core remains braced.

7. Stop what you're doing, and completely relax for 30 seconds to allow your brain a chance to integrate this work. Repeat the steps for leg movement one more time.

Arm Movement

1. Lie on your back with your knees bent and your feet on the floor slightly apart.

2. Place the fingers of your left and right hand on either side of your belly button, about one inch away from the center to feel your lower abdomen tighten when you brace. Gently rock your pelvis backward and forward a few times to find pelvic neutral.

3. Brace your core by lifting your pelvic floor, tightening your abdomen, and breathing to your belly button.

4. Slowly raise your right arm as high as you can above your head, and then bring it back to the starting position. Repeat this same motion with your left arm.

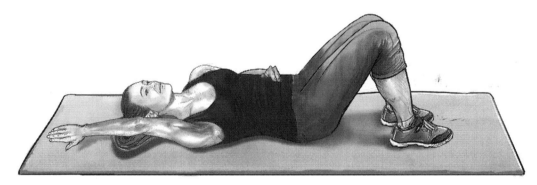

5. Slowly reach the right arm as far as you can across your left shoulder, and then bring it back to the starting position. Repeat this same motion with your left arm.

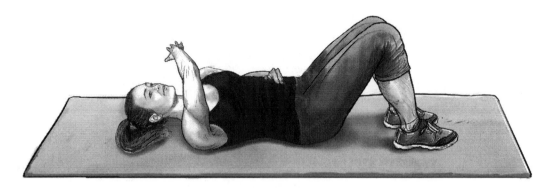

6. Repeat these motions three times while ensuring your pelvis and torso remain still and your core remains braced.

7. Stop what you're doing, and completely relax for 30 seconds to allow your body and brain a chance to integrate this work. Repeat the steps for arm movement one more time.

Combined Movement

1. Lie on your back with your knees bent and the soles of your feet on the floor slightly apart.

2. Place the fingers of your left and right hand on either side of your belly button, about one inch away from the center to feel your lower abdomen tighten when you brace. Gently rock your pelvis backward and forward a few times to find pelvic neutral.

3. Brace your core by lifting your pelvic floor, tightening your abdomen, and breathing to your belly button.

4. Slowly slide your right heel forward on the floor until your leg is straight, and then slide it back to the starting position. Simultaneously raise your left arm as high as you can above your head, and then bring it back to the starting position. Repeat these same motions with your opposite arm and leg.

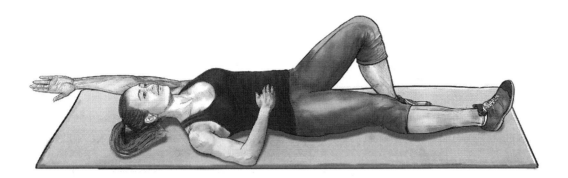

5. Slowly bring your right knee toward your chest, and then bring it back to the starting position. Simultaneously reach your left arm as far as you can across the right shoulder, and then bring it back to the starting position. Repeat these same motions with your opposite arm and leg.

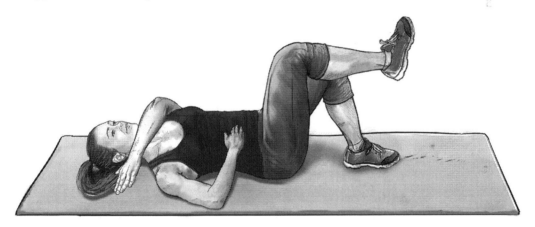

6. Repeat these motions three times while ensuring your pelvis and torso remain still and your core remains braced.

7. Stop what you're doing, and completely relax for 30 seconds to allow your body and brain a chance to integrate this work. Repeat the steps for combined movement one more time.

Now that you've mastered core bracing, you have the foundations to perform core strengthening exercises safely and effectively. You can also use core bracing with everyday movements to reduce pain, prevent injuries, and improve performance. Notice how you feel when you brace your core while standing up from sitting, bending over to pick up something, or carrying something heavy.

PART 3

Core Strengthening Exercises

Part 3 provides easy-to-follow instructions for over 25 at-home exercises using little or no equipment, with variations to match any fitness level. These exercises are based on scientific studies and my experience working with thousands of clients of all ages, weight, and fitness levels.

The exercises are divided into chapters based on the location of the muscles: front abdominals, side abdominals, back and shoulders, and hips and glutes. I've also included a chapter on important stretching exercises that work well with core exercises to improve posture, relieve pain, prevent injuries, and boost performance.

You might need some of the following equipment to increase the challenge of the exercises:

- a pair of one- to two-pound dumbbells
- a pair of one- to two-pound ankle weights (preferably the adjustable ankle weights that can each be adjusted between one to five pounds in one-pound increments)
- an open-loop resistance band

9. Front Abdominals

The exercises in this chapter target the muscles on the front of your torso, including the rectus abdominis and the transverse abdominis.

Dead Bug

The dead bug, so named because you look like a dead bug lying on its back, targets your abdominal muscles.

While this exercise is safe for most people, be careful if you have back or shoulder issues. Stop this exercise if it causes or increases pain in your back or shoulders.

Step-by-Step Instructions

1. Get into the starting position:

    *   Lie on your back with your knees bent and your feet flat on the floor.

    *   Lift your arms over your chest while keeping your elbows straight and your palms facing each other.

    *   Lift your feet off the floor with your hips and knees bent 90 degrees.

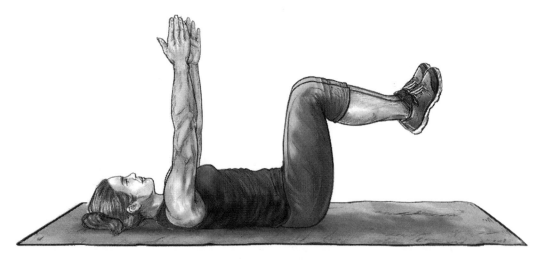

2. Brace your core by firing your pelvic floor and abdominal muscles while breathing to your belly button. Press your lower back to the floor and ensure it maintains contact with the floor throughout this exercise.

3. Begin exercising by slowly lowering your opposite arm and leg until they're a few inches above the floor. Hold for three seconds, and then slowly bring your arm and leg back to the starting position. Repeat with your opposite arm and leg.

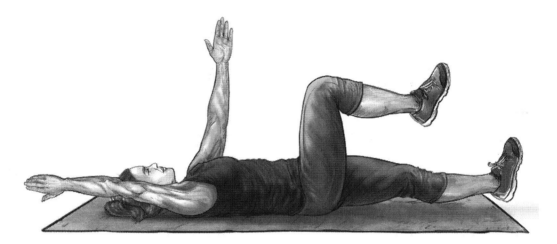

4. Perform 12 to 20 repetitions on each side.

Common Mistakes

*   **Moving too fast:** Since slowing down makes this exercise more effective, you want to strive for a pace of three seconds to lower your arm and leg, three seconds to hold, and three seconds to return your arm and leg to the starting position.

*   **Lifting your lower back off the floor:** Lifting your lower back off the floor increases strain in your lower back that can lead to pain. So press your lower back to the floor and ensure it maintains contact with the floor throughout this exercise. If you have difficulty doing this, you may need to start with a modification for beginners.

Modifications for Beginners

Dead Bug with Separate Limb Movement: Follow the same instructions for the dead bug, except lower one arm and then bring your arm back to the starting position.

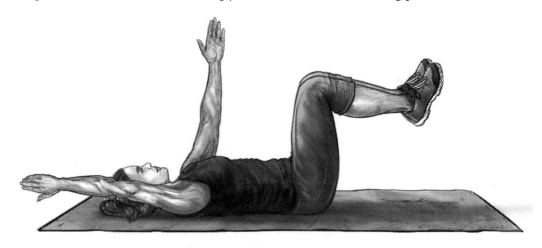

Lower your opposite leg and then bring your leg back to the starting position.

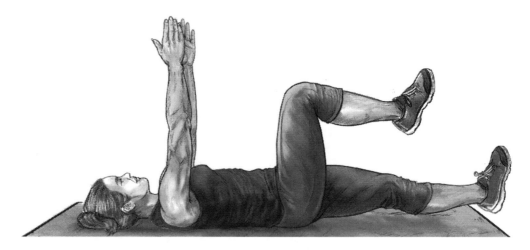

Repeat with your opposite arm and leg.

Variations to Challenge Yourself

Dead Bug with Weights: Follow the same instructions for the dead bug, except add ankle weights around each ankle and dumbbells in each hand. Start with one or two pounds, and gradually increase the resistance.

Static Trunk Lift

The static trunk lift is performed on your back and targets your upper abdominal muscles while also strengthening the deep muscles of your neck.

If you have neck or shoulder issues, be careful with this exercise. Stop this exercise if it causes or increases pain in your neck or shoulders.

Step-by-Step Instructions

1. Get into the starting position:
   - Lie on your back with your knees bent and your feet flat on the floor.
   - Lift your arms over your head with your elbows straight and your palms facing each other.
   - Lift your head one to two inches off the floor.

2. Brace your core by firing your pelvic floor and abdominal muscles while breathing to your belly button. Press your lower back to the floor, and ensure it maintains contact with the floor throughout this exercise.

3. Begin exercising by lifting your entire chest straight up toward the ceiling, without rounding your spine, until your entire upper back is one to two inches off the floor.

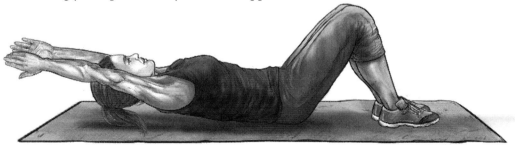

4. Hold for 30 to 60 seconds.

Common Mistakes

- **Forward or backward bending of your head:** Bringing your head too far forward or backward can strain your neck. To avoid this, lift your head one to two inches off the floor so your head is aligned with your torso. Not only will this protect your neck from injury, but you'll also get the deep muscles of your neck stronger.

- **Rounding your spine:** Rounding your spine forward like the motion that's made during sit-ups or crunches can cause strain on your lower back. So make sure to keep your spine straight by lifting your chest straight up toward the ceiling until your entire upper back is one to two inches off the floor. If you have difficulty keeping your spine straight or lifting your upper back off the floor, you may need to start with a modification for beginners.

Modifications for Beginners

Static Trunk Lift without Arms: Follow the same instructions for the static trunk lift, except keep your arms next to your body and your palms flat on the floor. This will reduce the resistance on your abdominal muscles from the weight of your arms.

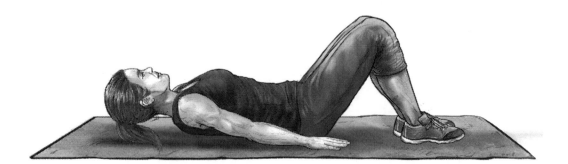

Variations to Challenge Yourself

Static Trunk Lift with Weights: Follow the same instructions for the static trunk lift, except add dumbbells in each hand. Start with one or two pounds, and gradually increase the resistance.

Static Leg Lift

The static leg lift is performed on your back and targets your lower abdominal muscles while also strengthening the deep muscles of your neck.

Be careful with this exercise if you have neck or lower back issues. Stop this exercise if it causes or increases pain in your neck or lower back.

Step-by-Step Instructions

1. Get into the starting position:

   - Lie on your back with your knees bent and your feet flat on the floor.
   - Place your arms next to your body with your palms flat on the floor.
   - Lift your feet off the floor with your hips and knees bent 90 degrees.

2. Brace your core by firing your pelvic floor and abdominal muscles while breathing to your belly button. Press your lower back to the floor, and ensure it maintains contact with the floor throughout this exercise. Lift your head one to two inches off the floor.

3. Begin exercising by slowly bringing both legs forward until your knees are straight and your heels are about two feet above the floor.

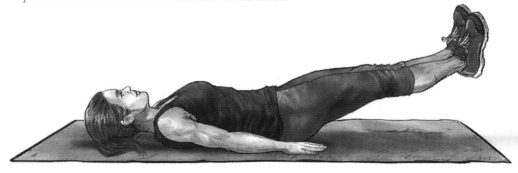

4. Hold for 30 to 60 seconds. End this exercise by first bringing both knees toward your chest and then placing your feet on the floor with your knees bent.

Common Mistakes

-   **Ending the exercise incorrectly:** If you end this exercise by releasing your feet directly to the floor, you can cause strain on your lower back. So make sure to end this exercise by first bringing both knees toward your chest and then placing your feet on the floor with your knees bent.

-   **Lifting your lower back off the floor:** Lifting your lower back off the floor increases strain in your lower back that can lead to pain. To avoid this, press your lower back to the floor and ensure it maintains contact with the floor throughout this exercise. If you have difficulty doing this, you may need to start with a modification for beginners.

Modifications for Beginners

Static Leg Lift with Knees Bent: Follow the same instructions for the static leg lift, except begin exercising in the starting position with your hips and knees bent 90 degrees. To increase the challenge of this modification, exercise with your legs halfway between the starting position and your knees straight with your heels two feet above the floor.

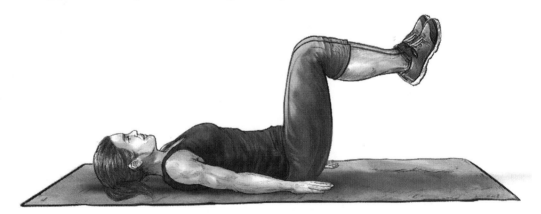

Variations to Challenge Yourself

Static Leg Lift with Weights: Follow the same instructions for the static leg lift, except add ankle weights around each ankle. Start with one or two pounds, and gradually increase the resistance.

Front Plank

The front plank is performed in a position similar to a push-up and targets your abdominal muscles.

If you have shoulder, elbow, or lower back issues, be careful with this exercise. Stop this exercise if it causes or increases pain in your shoulders, elbows, or back.

Step-by-Step Instructions

1. Get into the starting position:
   - Lie face down on the floor with your elbows directly under your shoulders, your forearms pointing forward, and your palms flat on the floor.
   - Place your feet hip-width apart with your toes and knees on the floor.
   - Align your head with your spine and keep your eyes looking down at the floor.

2. Brace your core by firing your pelvic floor and abdominal muscles while breathing to your belly button.

3. Begin exercising by lifting your torso and knees off the floor so that the entire length of your back is parallel to the floor. Your elbows, forearms, and toes should be the only parts of your body touching the floor.

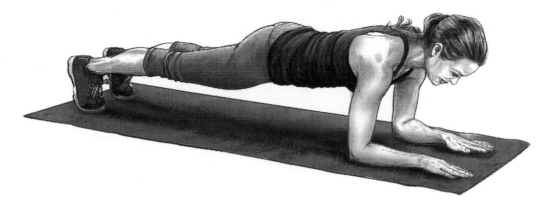

4. Hold for 30 to 60 seconds.

Common Mistakes

- **Allowing your hips to sag:** Your hips should remain in a straight line with your back and shoulders. If you have difficulty keeping your hips from sagging, you may need to start with a modification for beginners.

- **Tilting your head up:** Tilting your head up to look straight ahead or at the ceiling can put strain on your neck. So to avoid this, make sure your eyes are looking down at the floor and your head is aligned with your spine.

Modifications for Beginners

Front Plank on Knees: Follow the same instructions for the front plank, except keep your knees and toes on the floor. Increase the challenge of this modification by moving your knees farther back so there's a larger space between your elbows and knees.

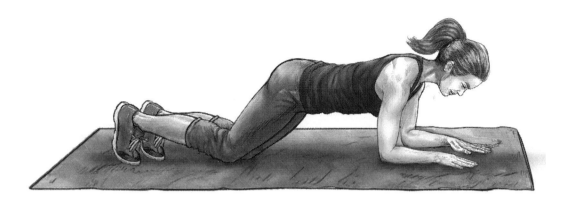

Variations to Challenge Yourself

Front Plank with Leg Lift: Follow the same instructions for the front plank, except lift one leg six to eight inches off the floor. Hold for 15 to 30 seconds, then repeat on the opposite leg.

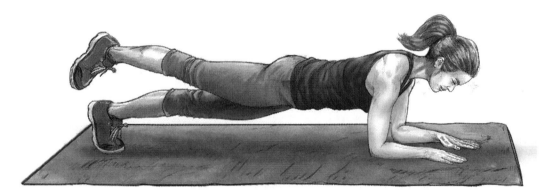

Front Plank with Arm Lift: Follow the same instructions for the front plank, except lift one arm straight out in front of you. Hold for 15 to 30 seconds, then repeat on the opposite arm.

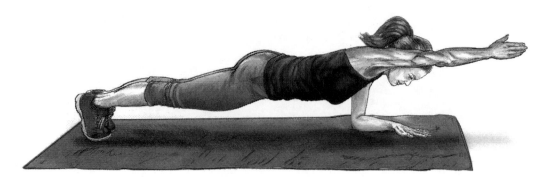

Front Plank with Opposite Lift: Follow the same instructions for the front plank, except simultaneously lift one leg six to eight inches off the floor and the opposite arm straight out in front of you. Hold for 15 to 30 seconds, then repeat on the opposite arm and leg.

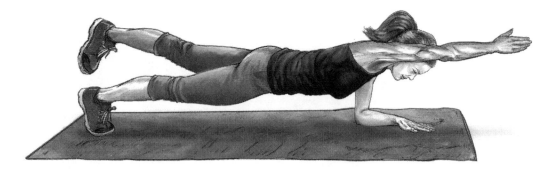

10. Side Abdominals

The exercises in this chapter target the muscles on the sides of your torso, including the internal obliques and external obliques.

Anti-Rotation Wall Press

The anti-rotation wall press is performed while standing in front of a wall corner and targets your oblique muscles on the sides of your torso.

Although this exercise is safe for most people, be careful if you have wrist or shoulder issues. Stop this exercise if it causes or increases pain in your wrists or shoulders.

Step-by-Step Instructions

1. Get into the starting position:

    - Stand a few feet in front of a wall corner with your arms straight out in front of you at about shoulder height and your fingers together.

    - Place the back of your right hand against the wall with your arms centered in front of your body.

    - Place your feet hip-width apart with a slight bend in the knees.

2. Brace your core by firing your pelvic floor and abdominal muscles while breathing to your belly button.

3. Begin exercising by using both arms to push the back of your right hand against the wall as firmly as you can for three seconds, while your arms and torso should remain motionless. Stop pushing for three seconds while keeping your hands in place. Alternate between pushing for three seconds and not pushing for three seconds.

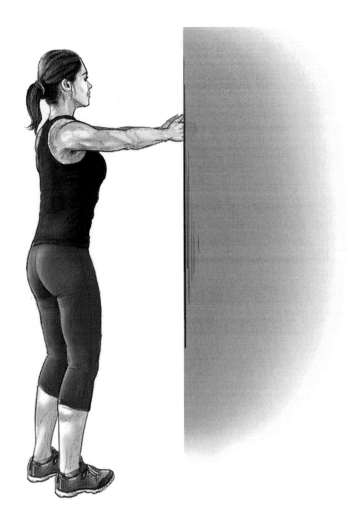

4. Perform 12 to 20 repetitions, then repeat on the opposite side.

Common Mistakes

*   **Improper hand placement on the wall:** Proper placement of your hands on the wall is important for getting the best results from this exercise. You want to make sure your arms are about shoulder height, with your elbows straight and only the part of your hand that's below the wrist touching the wall.

- **Movement in your arms or torso while pushing:** Because movement in your arms or torso while pushing will make this exercise less effective, you want to make sure to brace your core to prevent this. If you have difficulty doing this, you may need to start with a modification for beginners.

Modifications for Beginners

Wide-Stance Anti-Rotation Press: Follow the same instructions for the anti-rotation wall press, except widen your feet to about three feet apart.

Variations to Challenge Yourself

Narrow-Stance Anti-Rotation Press: Follow the same instructions for the anti-rotation wall press, except place your feet together.

Resistance Band Anti-Rotation Press: This variation of the anti-rotation wall press requires an elastic resistance band wrapped around or fastened to a stable anchor point about chest high.

1. Get into the starting position:

   - Grasp the free end of the resistance band firmly in both hands and hold your hands against your chest.

   - Sidestep away from the anchor point, with the anchor point to one side of your body, until the band becomes tight. Keep your legs hip-width apart and your knees slightly bent.

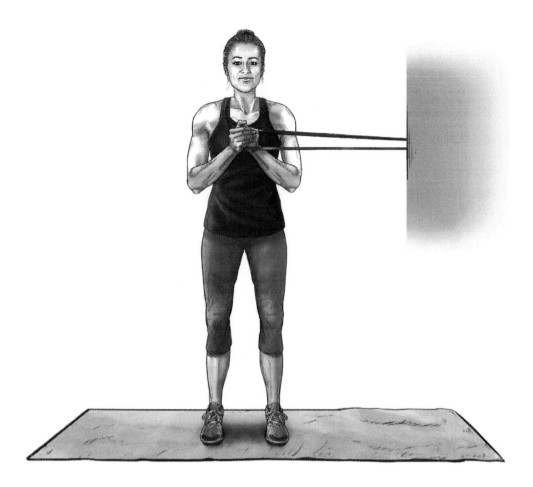

2. Brace your core by firing your pelvic floor and abdominal muscles while breathing to your belly button.

3. Begin exercising by pressing the band away from your chest until your arms are straight and hold this position for three seconds while your arms and torso remain motionless. Bring the band back to your chest and hold this position for three seconds. Alternate between holding the band away from your chest for three seconds and holding the band against your chest for three seconds.

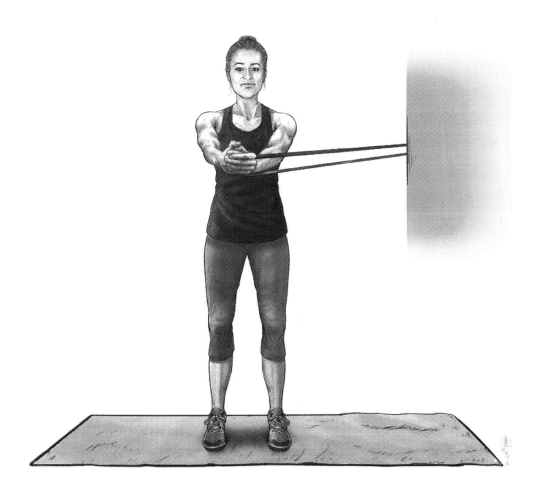

4. Perform 12 to 20 repetitions, then repeat on the opposite side.

Oblique Half Twist

The oblique half twist is performed on your back and targets your oblique muscles on the sides of your torso.

Avoid this exercise if you have a history of spine surgery and stop this exercise if it causes or increases pain in your back or hips.

Step-by-Step Instructions

1. Get into the starting position:

    - Lie on your back with your knees bent and your feet flat on the floor.

    - Spread your arms to the sides of your body at shoulder height, with your palms flat on the floor.

    - Lift your feet off the floor with your hips and knees bent 90 degrees.

2. Brace your core by firing your pelvic floor and abdominal muscles while breathing to your belly button.

3. Begin exercising by slowly lowering your legs toward the floor on one side of your body with your feet together. Stop when your legs are halfway to the floor and hold this position for three seconds.

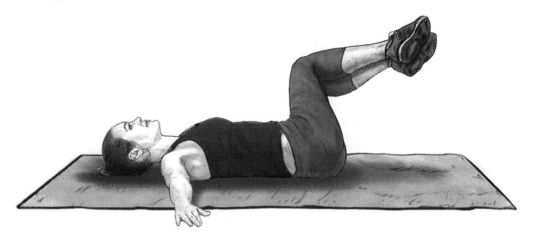

Slowly bring your legs back to the center, then repeat on the opposite side.

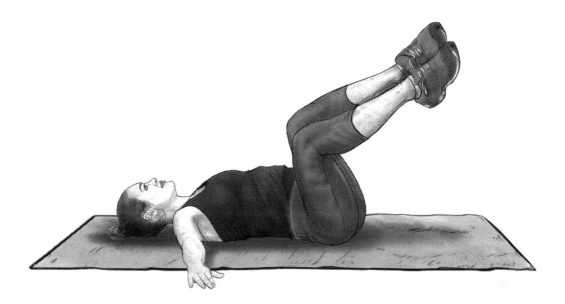

4. Perform 12 to 20 repetitions on both sides.

Common Mistakes

- **Lowering your legs too much:** Lowering your legs too much toward the floor can strain your back. So make sure to stop the motion when your legs are halfway to the floor.

- **Moving too fast:** Since slowing down will make this exercise more effective, you should strive for a pace of three seconds to lower your legs, three seconds to hold, and three seconds to return the legs to the starting position.

- **Not keeping your feet together:** Separating your feet will make this exercise less effective. So make sure to keep your feet together throughout this exercise.

- **Letting your shoulders lift off the floor:** To get the best results from this exercise, you want to make sure your shoulders stay glued to the floor.

Modifications for Beginners

Oblique Quarter Twist: Follow the same instructions for the oblique half twist, except reduce your range of motion by lowering your legs only a quarter of the way to each side.

Variations to Challenge Yourself

Oblique Half Twist with Weights: Follow the same instructions for the oblique half twist, except add ankle weights around each ankle. Start with one or two pounds, and gradually increase the resistance.

Side Body Lift

The side body lift, which targets your oblique muscles on the sides of your torso, is performed on your side while lying on a yoga bolster or thick pillow.

While this exercise is safe for most people, be careful if you have neck or back issues. Stop this exercise if it causes or increases pain in your neck or back.

Step-by-Step Instructions

1. Get into the starting position:
   - Lie on one side of your body on top of a yoga bolster or thick pillow that's centered with your belly button.
   - Keep your torso and legs in a straight line with your feet stacked on top of each other.
   - Place your bottom arm on the floor, straight out in front of your chest for balance, while you extend your top arm toward the ceiling.

2. Brace your core by firing your pelvic floor and abdominal muscles while breathing to your belly button.

3. Begin exercising by lifting your shoulders and both legs a few inches off the floor, so your entire body is in a straight line from head to toes.

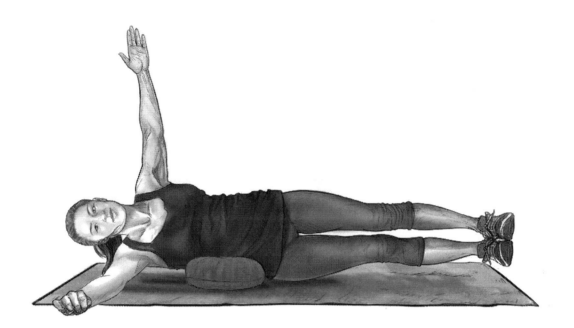

4. Hold for 30 to 60 seconds, then repeat on the opposite side.

Common Mistakes

- **Placing too much weight on your bottom arm:** Since placing too much weight on your bottom arm will make this exercise less effective, you want to ensure your bottom arm is lightly touching the floor for balance.

- **Lifting your shoulders or legs too high:** Lifting your shoulders or legs too high will increase strain on your spine. To avoid this, make sure your entire body is in a straight line from head to toes.

- **Rotating your body forward or backward:** Rotating your body forward or backward will prevent you from working the correct muscles on the sides of your torso. So make sure that your shoulders, hips, and legs are stacked on top of each other throughout this exercise.

Modifications for Beginners

Modified Side Body Lift: Your starting position will be the same as the side body lift, except you want to place your top arm along the side of your body. Begin exercising by lifting your shoulders and your top leg while keeping your bottom leg on the floor.

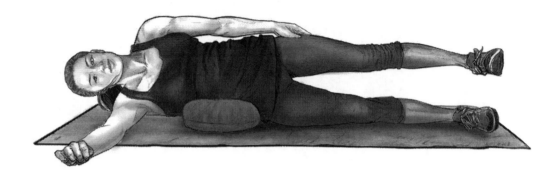

Variations to Challenge Yourself

Side Body Lift with Weights: Follow the same instructions for the side body lift, except hold a dumbbell in your top hand. Start with one or two pounds, and gradually increase the resistance.

Side Plank

The side plank is performed on your side and targets your oblique muscles on the sides of your torso.

Be careful with this exercise if you have shoulder or elbow issues. Stop this exercise if it causes or increases pain in your shoulders or elbows.

Step-by-Step Instructions

1. Get into the starting position:

    - Lie on one side of your body with your torso and legs in a straight line and your feet stacked on top of each other.

    - Place your bottom elbow on the floor directly under your shoulder.

    - Ensure your top hand is resting on your waist.

2. Brace your core by firing your pelvic floor and abdominal muscles while breathing to your belly button.

3. Begin exercising by lifting your body off the floor so that your entire body is in a straight line from head to toe. Your bottom elbow and foot should be supporting your entire body weight.

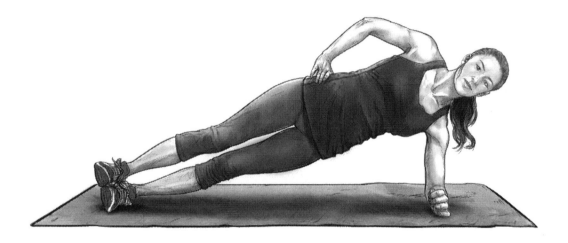

4. Hold for 30 to 60 seconds, then repeat on the opposite side.

Common Mistakes

- **Allowing your hips to sag:** Your hips should remain in a straight line between your knees and shoulders. If you have difficulty keeping your hips from sagging, you may need to start with a modification for beginners.

- **Rotating your body forward or backward:** Because rotating your body forward or backward will prevent you from working the correct muscles on the sides of your torso, you want to make sure that your shoulders, hips, and legs are stacked on top of each other throughout this exercise.

Modifications for Beginners

Side Plank on Knees: Follow the same instructions for the side plank, except bend both knees 90 degrees and keep your knees on the floor when you lift your body off the floor.

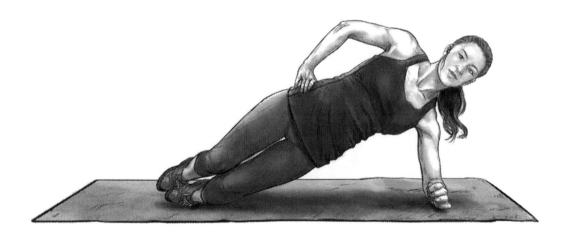

Variations to Challenge Yourself

Side Plank with Weights: Follow the same instructions for the side plank, except place a dumbbell on your top waist and hold it in place with your top hand. Start with one pound, and gradually increase the resistance.

Single Leg Stance

The single leg stance, which targets your oblique muscles and improves your balance, is performed while standing with a dumbbell in one hand.

This exercise is safe for most people, but be careful if your balance is very poor. In case you need to hold on to something to prevent yourself from falling, perform this exercise in front of a kitchen counter or a sturdy table.

Step-by-Step Instructions

Use a 10-pound weight for this exercise or a backpack filled with canned goods of equivalent weight.

1. Get into the starting position:

    *   Stand tall with your feet together and your eyes looking straight forward.

    *   Hold the weight or backpack in one hand.

    *   Place your other hand on your waist.

2. Brace your core by firing your pelvic floor and abdominal muscles while breathing to your belly button.

3. Begin exercising by lifting the leg that's on the same side as the arm holding the weight until your hip and knee are bent 90 degrees. Make sure you're standing tall and your eyes are looking straight forward.

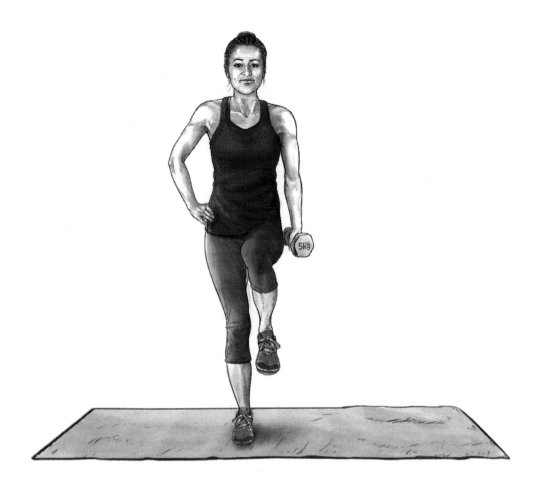

4. Hold for 30 to 60 seconds, then repeat on the opposite side.

Common Mistakes

- **Leg coming down:** If your leg keeps coming down to the ground because you're losing balance, you may need to start with a modification for beginners.

- **Bending your torso:** Although motion of the torso is normal with balancing exercises, too much bending forward, backward, or to the sides will increase strain on your back. Try to keep your torso as motionless as possible throughout this exercise. If you have difficulty doing this, you may need to start with a modification for beginners.

Modifications for Beginners

Single Leg Stance without Weight: If you're having trouble with balance, perform the single leg stance without a weight. If you're still having trouble with balance, try lifting your leg a few inches off the floor.

Variations to Challenge Yourself

Single Leg Stance with Heavier Weight: Follow the same instructions for the single leg stance, except use a heavier weight.

Single Leg Stance with Eyes Closed: Follow the same instructions for the single leg stance, except with your eyes closed. Increase the challenge of this variation by using a heavier weight.

Single Leg Stance on a Pillow: Follow the same instructions for the single leg stance, except stand on a pillow, foam balance pad, or Bosu ball to challenge your balance. Increase the challenge of this variation by closing your eyes and/or using a heavier weight.

11. Back and Shoulders

The exercises in this chapter target the muscles of the back and shoulders: the lumbar multifidus, paraspinals, latissimus dorsi, and trapezius.

Bird Dog

The bird dog, so named because you look like a bird dog pointing at a bird, is performed on all fours and targets your back and glute (butt) muscles.

Stop this exercise if it causes or increases pain in your back or shoulders.

Step-by-Step Instructions

1. Get into the starting position:

    - Get on all fours on the floor with your knees hip-width apart directly under your hips and your hands shoulder-width apart directly under your shoulders.

    - Ensure your back and head are parallel to the floor.

    - Look down at the floor.

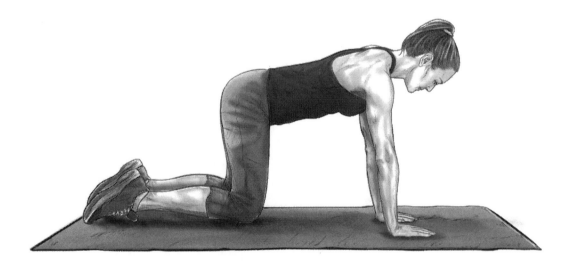

2. Brace your core by firing your pelvic floor and abdominal muscles while breathing to your belly button.

3. Begin exercising by slowly lifting one arm out in front of you with your thumb pointed up, while simultaneously lifting your opposite leg behind you until your arm and leg are aligned with your torso. Hold for three seconds, and then slowly bring your arm and leg back to the starting position. Repeat with your opposite arm and leg.

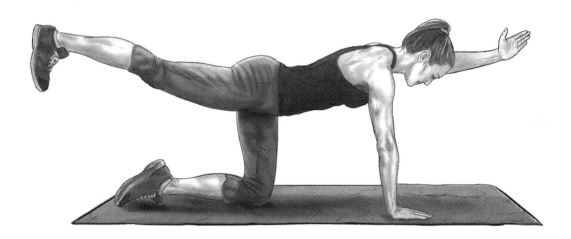

4. Perform 12 to 20 repetitions on each side.

Common Mistakes

- **Motion in your torso:** To reduce strain on your back, you want to avoid moving your torso. So make sure to brace your core so your torso remains motionless as you lift and lower your arms and legs. If you have difficulty preventing motion in your torso, you may need to start with a modification for beginners.

- **Arching your lower back:** Avoid arching your lower back by bracing your core when lifting your arms and legs to prevent strain on your back. If you have difficulty preventing your lower back from arching, you may need to start with a modification for beginners.

- **Tilting your head up:** Since tilting your head up to look straight ahead or at the ceiling can put strain on your neck, make sure you're looking down at the floor with your head in a neutral position.

- **Moving too fast:** You don't want to move too fast. Strive for a pace of three seconds to lift your opposite arm and leg, three seconds to hold, and three seconds to return your arm and leg to the starting position.

Modifications for Beginners

Bird Dog with Arms Only: Follow the same instructions for the bird dog, except alternate between lifting the left and right arm without lifting the legs.

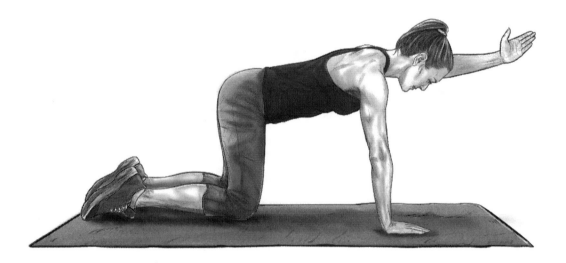

Bird Dog with Legs Only: This modification is more challenging than the bird dog with arms only. Follow the same instructions for the bird dog, except alternate between lifting the left and right leg without lifting the arms.

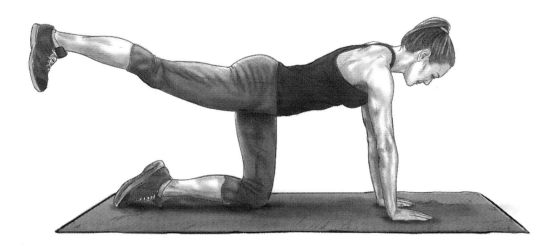

Variations to Challenge Yourself

Bird Dog with Weights: Follow the same instructions for the bird dog, except add ankle weights around each ankle and dumbbells in each hand. Start with one or two pounds and gradually increase the resistance.

Modified Superman

The modified superman is performed on your stomach and targets your back and glute (butt) muscles. This version of the superman is "modified" to avoid extreme arching of the lower back that the superman exercise typically entails.

Stop this exercise if it causes or increases pain in your back or shoulders.

Step-by-Step Instructions

1. Get into the starting position:

   - Lie on your stomach with your arms extended over your head shoulder-width apart and your legs straight with your feet hip-width apart.

   - Make sure your forehead, arms, and legs are resting on the floor.

2. Brace your core by firing your pelvic floor and abdominal muscles while breathing to your belly button.

3. Begin exercising by squeezing your butt muscles and slowly lifting your forehead, arms, and legs three to six inches off the floor while keeping your arms and legs straight. Your chest and pelvis should remain on the floor, and your eyes should be looking straight down.

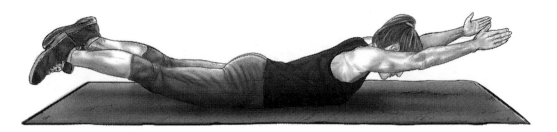

4. Hold for 30 to 60 seconds.

Common Mistakes

- **Bending your arms or legs:** Because bending your elbows or knees while lifting will make this exercise less effective, you want to make sure to keep your arms and legs straight while lifting to get the best results from this exercise. If you have difficulty preventing your arms and legs from bending, you may need to start with a modification for beginners.

- **Arching your lower back:** Avoid arching your lower back by bracing your core when lifting your arms and legs to prevent strain on your back. If you have difficulty preventing your lower back from arching, you may need to start with a modification for beginners.

- **Tilting your head up:** Tilting your head up to look straight ahead or at the ceiling can put strain on your neck. So make sure you're looking down at the floor with your head in a neutral position to protect your neck.

- **Holding your breath:** Try to avoid holding your breath with this exercise to get the best results.

Modifications for Beginners

Modified Superman with Arms Only: Follow the same instructions for the modified superman, except lift both arms without lifting the legs.

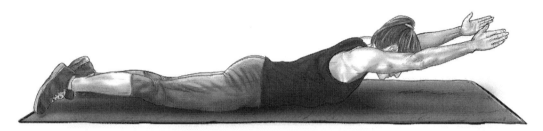

Modified Superman with Legs Only: This modification is more challenging than the modified superman with arms only. Follow the same instructions for the modified superman, except lift both legs without lifting the arms.

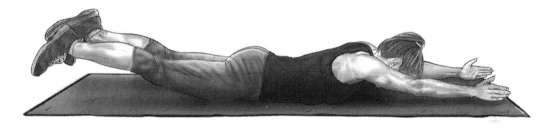

Variations to Challenge Yourself

Modified Superman with Weights: Follow the same instructions for the modified superman, except add ankle weights around each ankle and dumbbells in each hand. Start with one or two pounds, and gradually increase the resistance.

TUY Arm Lift

The TUY arm lift, which targets your middle and upper back muscles, gets its name from the shape you make with your arms that resemble the letters *T*, *U*, and *Y*.

Stop this exercise if it causes or increases pain in your back or shoulders.

Step-by-Step Instructions

1. Get into the starting position:

   - Lie face down on your stomach with your legs straight and your arms forming the shape of the letter *T* with your arms on the floor and your thumbs pointed up.

   - Squeeze your shoulder blades together and lower them down.

   - Lift your forehead one inch off the floor with your eyes looking straight down.

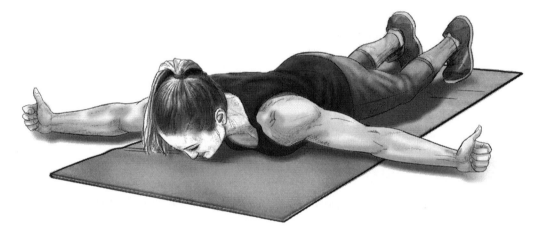

2. Brace your core by firing your pelvic floor and abdominal muscles while breathing to your belly button.

3. Begin exercising by lifting your arms three to six inches off the floor while keeping your arms straight.

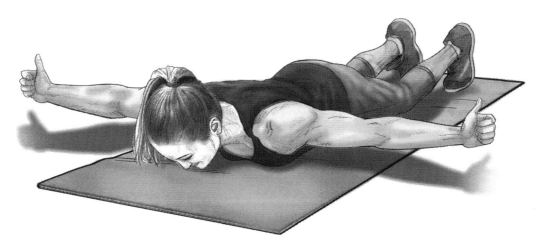

Hold this position for three seconds, and then slowly bend your elbows until your arms form the letter *U*.

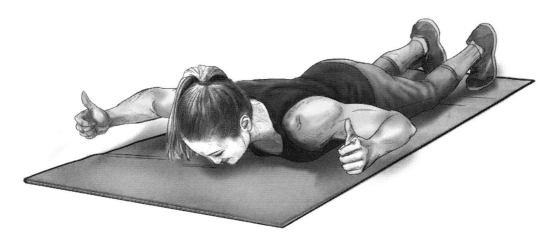

Hold this position for three seconds, then slowly straighten your arms overhead until they form the letter *Y*.

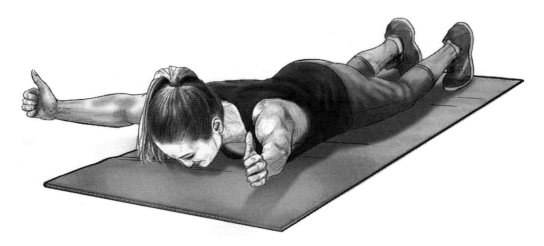

Hold this position for three seconds, then slowly sweep your arms toward your sides to form the letter *T*.

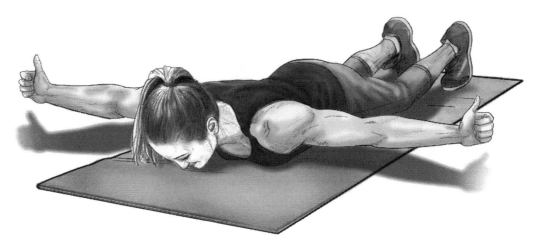

Hold this position for three seconds.

4. Perform 12 to 20 repetitions.

Common Mistakes

- **Lowering your arms to the floor:** Your arms should remain three to six inches off the floor throughout this exercise to get the best results. If you have difficulty keeping your arms lifted, you may need to start with a modification for beginners.

- **Tilting your head up:** Since tilting your head up to look straight ahead or at the ceiling can put strain on your neck, make sure you look down at the floor with your head in a neutral position.

- **Moving too fast:** Slowing it down will make this exercise more effective. So strive for a pace of three seconds in each position and three seconds to move into the next position.

- **Thumbs not pointing up:** Keep your thumbs pointed up so you don't injure your shoulders.

Modifications for Beginners

T Arm Lift: Form the shape of the letter *T* with your arms on the floor and your thumbs pointed up.

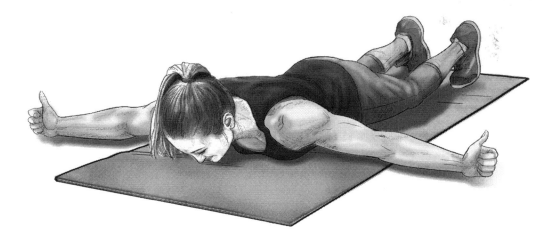

Begin exercising by slowly lifting your arms three to six inches off the floor.

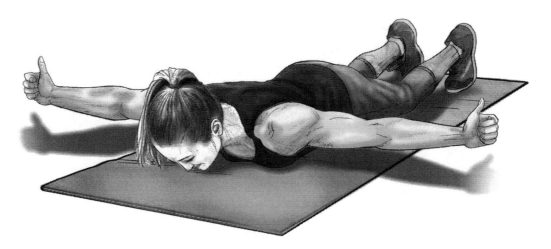

Hold for three seconds, then slowly bring your arms back to the floor. Perform 12 to 20 repetitions. To increase the challenge of this modification, add one- or two-pound dumbbells in each hand and gradually increase the resistance.

U Arm Lift: This modification is more challenging than the T arm lift for most people. Form the shape of the letter *U* with your arms on the floor and your thumbs pointed up.

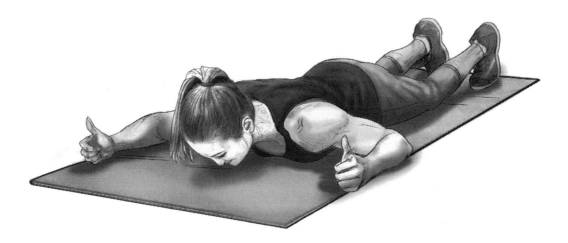

Begin exercising by slowly lifting your arms three to six inches off the floor, while ensuring your wrists and elbows are lifted the same height.

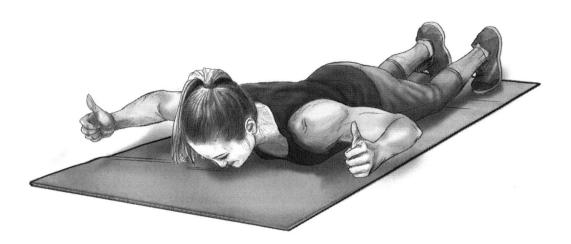

Hold for three seconds, then slowly bring your arms back to the floor. Perform 12 to 20 repetitions. To increase the challenge of this modification, add one- or two-pound dumbbells in each hand and gradually increase the resistance.

Y Arm Lift: This modification is more challenging than the U arm lift for most people. Form the shape of the letter *Y* with your arms on the floor and your thumbs pointed up.

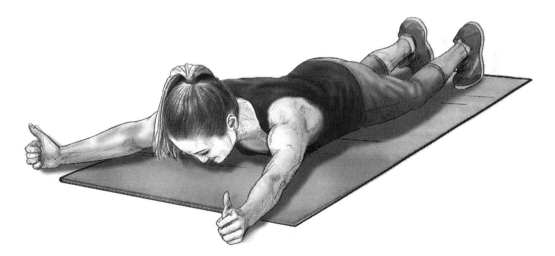

Begin exercising by slowly lifting your arms three to six inches off the floor.

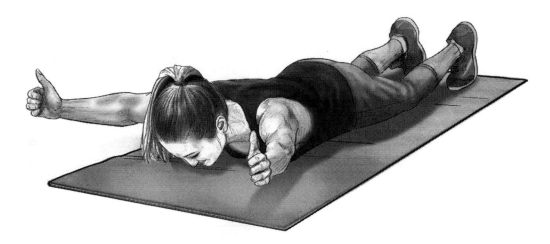

Hold for three seconds, then slowly bring your arms back to the floor. Perform 12 to 20 repetitions. To increase the challenge of this modification, add one- or two-pound dumbbells in each hand and gradually increase the resistance.

Variations to Challenge Yourself

TUY Arm Lift with Weights: Follow the same instructions for the TUY arm lift, except add dumbbells in each hand. Start with one or two pounds, and gradually increase the resistance.

Floor Push

The floor push, which is performed on your back, targets your latissimus dorsi muscle and strengthens the deep muscles of your neck.

Stop this exercise if it causes or increases pain in your neck or shoulders.

Step-by-Step Instructions

1. Get into the starting position:

    *   Lie on your back with your knees bent and your feet flat on the floor. Tuck your elbows against your torso and bend them at a 90-degree angle.

    *   Lower your shoulders down and lift your head one to two inches off the floor.

    *   Lift your feet off the floor with your hips and knees bent 90 degrees.

2. Brace your core by firing your pelvic floor and abdominal muscles while breathing to your belly button.

3. Begin exercising by pushing the back of your arms against the floor to lift your upper back and shoulders one to two inches off the floor while keeping your torso in a straight line.

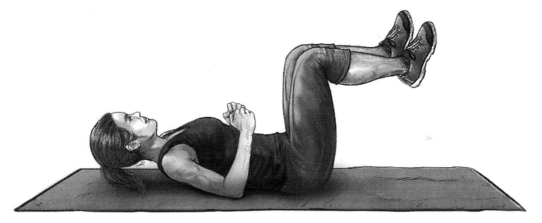

4. Hold for 30 to 60 seconds.

Common Mistakes

*   **Forward or backward bending of your head:** Bringing your head too far forward or backward can strain your neck. To avoid this, lift your head one to two inches off the floor so your head is aligned with your torso. Not only will this protect your neck from injury, but you'll also get the deep muscles of your neck stronger.

- **Forward or backward bending of your torso:** Bending your torso forward or backward will make this exercise less effective. So make sure to keep your torso straight to get the best results. If you have difficulty keeping your torso straight, you may need to start with a modification for beginners.

Modifications for Beginners

Wall Push: Follow the same instructions for the floor push, except stand with your back against a wall and your heels one foot away from the wall. Make this modification more challenging by placing your heels two feet away from the wall.

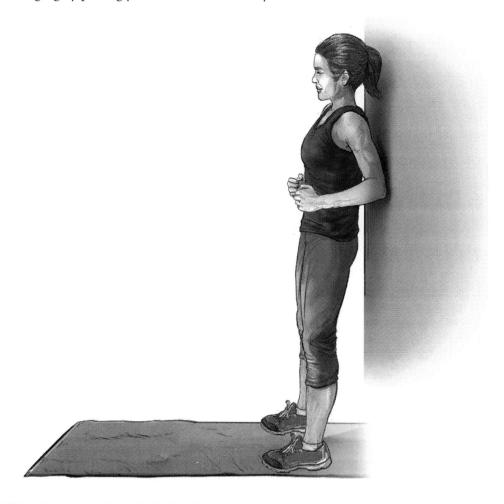

Variations to Challenge Yourself

Floor Push with Weights: Follow the same instructions for the floor push, except place an ankle weight across your chest. Start with one or two pounds, and gradually increase the resistance.

12. Hips and Glutes

The exercises in this chapter target the muscles of the hips and glutes: the gluteus maximus, hamstrings, hip abductors, and hip adductors.

Hip Raise

The hip raise is performed on your back and targets your glutes (butt).

Stop this exercise if it causes or increases pain in your back.

Step-by-Step Instructions

1. Get into the starting position:

    • Lie on your back with your knees bent and your feet flat on the floor hip-width distance apart.

    • Rest your arms next to your body with your palms flat on the floor.

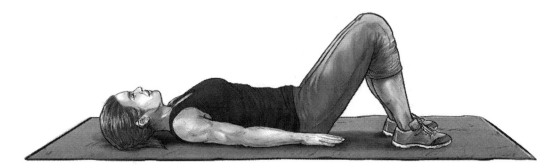

2. Brace your core by firing your pelvic floor and abdominal muscles while breathing to your belly button.

3. Begin exercising by raising your hips to create a straight line from your knees to your shoulders. Your knees should be bent 90 degrees with your hips lifted.

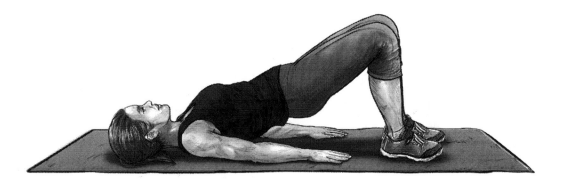

4. Hold for 30 to 60 seconds.

Common Mistakes

- **Knees not bent 90 degrees:** Bending your knees too much will not work your glutes effectively, while not bending your knees enough will cause strain on your lower back. So make sure your knees are bent 90 degrees with your hips lifted to get the best results from this exercise.

- **Raising your hips too high:** Raising your hips too high will hyperextend your lower back and cause strain. To avoid this, brace your core and ensure your shoulders, hips, and knees form a straight line.

- **Allowing your hips to sag:** Your hips should remain in a straight line between your knees and shoulders. If you have difficulty keeping your hips from sagging, you may need to start with a modification for beginners.

Modifications for Beginners

Repeated Hip Raise: Follow the same instructions for the hip raise, except repeatedly raise and lower your hips for 12 to 20 repetitions without holding in between.

Variations to Challenge Yourself

Single Leg Hip Raise: Follow the same instructions for the hip raise, except raise your hips on a single leg by lifting and extending one leg. Hold for 30 to 60 seconds, then repeat on the opposite side.

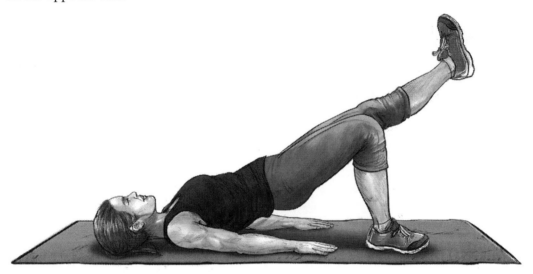

Heel Bridge with Marches

The heel bridge with marches is performed on your back and targets your hamstring muscles on the back of your thighs. You'll need a chair, bench, or stool that's about one to two feet high for this exercise.

If you have a hamstring injury, avoid this exercise. Stop this exercise if it causes or increases pain in your hamstrings or back.

Step-by-Step Instructions

1. Get into the starting position:

   - Lie on your back with your knees bent 90 degrees and the back of your heels hip-width apart on a chair, bench, or stool.

   - Rest your arms next to your body with your palms flat on the floor.

   - Brace your core by firing your pelvic floor and abdominal muscles while breathing to your belly button.

   - Push down on the back of your heels to raise your hips until you create a straight line from your knees to your shoulders.

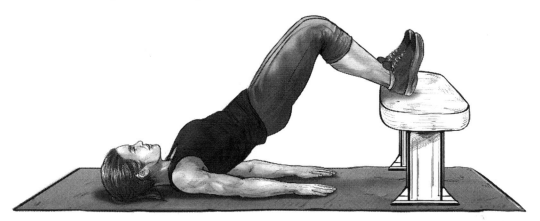

2. Begin exercising by lifting one heel off the chair for three seconds while keeping your hips lifted and level.

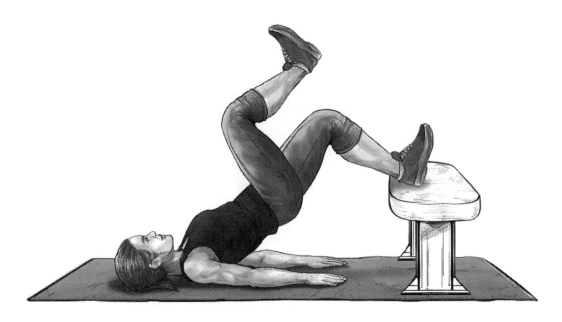

Place your heel back on the chair and repeat with your opposite leg.

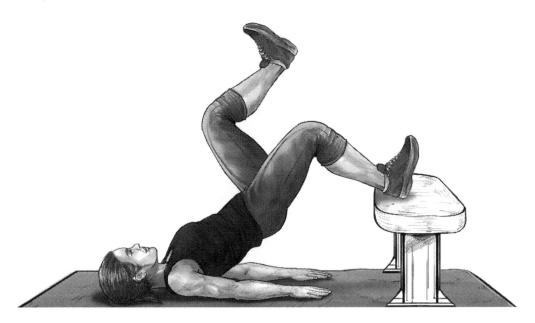

3. Perform 12 to 20 repetitions on each side.

Common Mistakes

- **Allowing your hips to sag:** Your hips should remain in a straight line between your knees and shoulders. If you have difficulty keeping your hips from sagging, you may need to start with a modification for beginners.

- **Hips not remaining level:** Your hips should remain level with each other as you alternate lifting the right and left leg. If you have difficulty keeping your hips level, you may need to start with a modification for beginners.

Modifications for Beginners

Double Leg Heel Bridge: Follow the same instructions for the heel bridge with marches, except on both legs without the marches. Push down on the back of your heels to raise your hips until you create a straight line from your knees to your shoulders. Hold for 30 to 60 seconds.

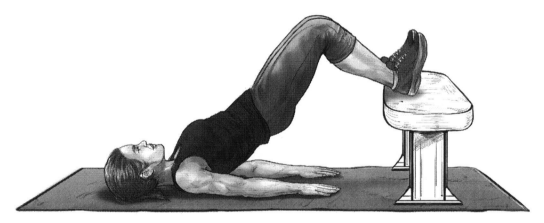

Variations to Challenge Yourself

Single Leg Heel Bridge: Follow the same instructions for the heel bridge with marches, except on a single leg without the marches. Push down on the back of your heels to raise your hips until you create a straight line from your knees to your shoulders. Lift and straighten one leg off the chair. Hold for 30 to 60 seconds, then repeat on the opposite side.

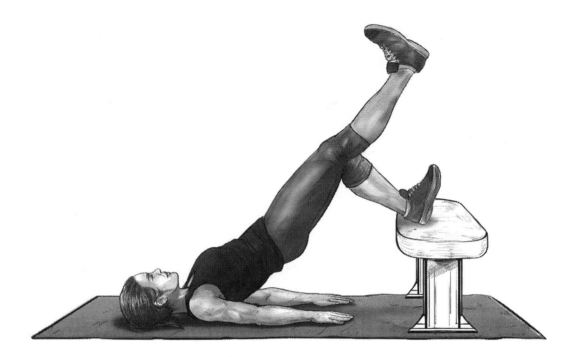

Side-Lying Leg Lift

The side-lying leg lift is performed on your side and targets your hip abductor muscles on your outer hip.

This exercise is safe for most people, but be careful if you have hip issues. Stop this exercise if it causes or increases pain in your hips.

Step-by-Step Instructions

1. Get into the starting position:

    *   Lie on one side of your body with your torso and legs in a straight line and your feet stacked on top of each other.

    *   Rest your head on your bottom arm and place the hand of your top arm on the floor in front of you for balance.

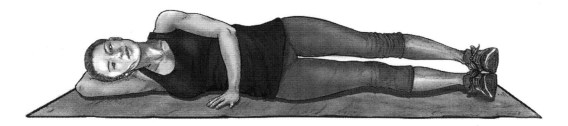

2. Brace your core by firing your pelvic floor and abdominal muscles while breathing to your belly button.

3. Begin exercising by slowly lifting your top leg two to three feet, pausing for a second at the top, and then slowly lowering it back to the starting position. Make sure to keep your top knee straight and your toes pointed forward throughout this exercise.

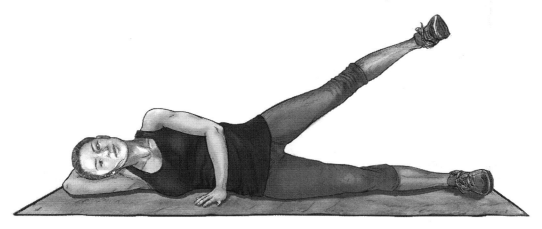

4. Perform 12 to 20 repetitions, then repeat on the opposite side.

Common Mistakes

Each of the mistakes below will make the side-lying leg lift less effective by reducing the work on the hip abductor muscles. If you have difficulty with any of them, you may need to start with a modification for beginners.

- **Pointing your toes up:** Make sure to keep your toes pointed straight forward while lifting your leg.

- **Bending your knee:** Make sure to tighten your thigh muscles to keep your top knee completely straight while lifting your leg.

- **Lifting your leg forward:** If you lift your leg forward, it will not work the correct muscles on your outer hip. So make sure to lift your leg straight up and straight down throughout this exercise.

- **Rotating your body backward:** If your body is rotated backward during this exercise, it'll prevent you from working the correct muscles on your outer hip. Make sure that your shoulders, hips, and legs are stacked on top of each other throughout this exercise.

Modifications for Beginners

Bent-Knee Side-Lying Leg Lift: Follow the same instructions for the side-lying leg lift, except bend your top knee 90 degrees in the starting position.

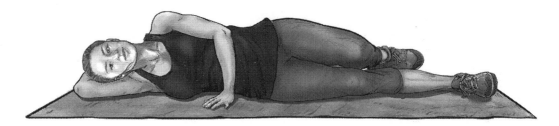

Lift and lower your top leg about one to two feet high with your knee bent in this position.

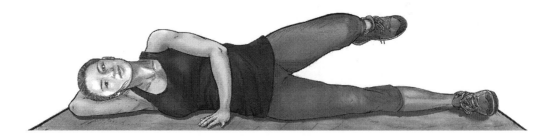

Variations to Challenge Yourself

Side-Lying Leg Lift with Weights: Follow the same instructions for the side-lying leg lift, except add an ankle weight around the ankle of your top leg. Start with one or two pounds, and gradually increase the resistance.

Single Leg Tuck

The single leg tuck is performed while lying on your side and targets your hip abductor muscles on your outer hip.

This exercise is safe for most people, but be careful if you have hip issues. Stop this exercise if it causes or increases pain in your hips.

Step-by-Step Instructions

1. Get into the starting position:

   - Lie on one side of your body with your torso and legs in a straight line and your feet stacked on top of each other.

   - Rest your head on your bottom arm and place the hand of your top arm on the floor in front of you for balance.

   - Lift your top leg hip-width apart from your bottom leg.

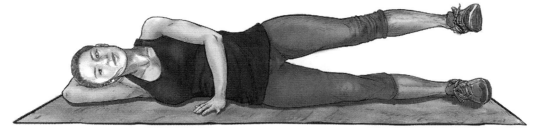

2. Brace your core by firing your pelvic floor and abdominal muscles while breathing to your belly button.

3. Begin exercising by slowly bringing your top leg forward in a tucking motion until your top hip and knee are bent 90 degrees.

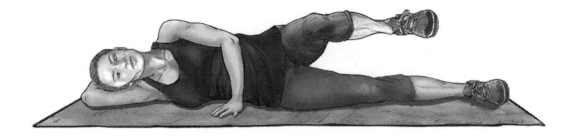

Hold for three seconds, then slowly bring your leg back to the starting position while keeping your legs hip-width apart.

4. Perform 12 to 20 repetitions, then repeat on the opposite side.

Common Mistakes

Each of the mistakes below will make the single leg tuck a less effective exercise by reducing the work on the hip abductor muscles. If you have difficulty with any of them, you may need to start with a modification for beginners.

- **Lifting your top leg too high:** Make sure to keep your legs hip-width apart throughout this exercise.

- **Dropping your knee:** Make sure to keep your legs hip-width apart throughout this exercise.

- **Rotating your body backward:** If your body is rotated backward during this exercise, it'll prevent you from working the correct muscles on your outer hip. Make sure that your shoulders and hips are stacked on top of each other throughout this exercise.

- **Moving too fast:** You want to strive for a pace of three seconds to bring your leg forward, three seconds to hold, and three seconds to return the leg to the starting position.

Modifications for Beginners

Single Leg Tuck Lift: Begin in the same starting position for the single leg tuck, except with your top hip and knee bent 90 degrees and resting on the floor.

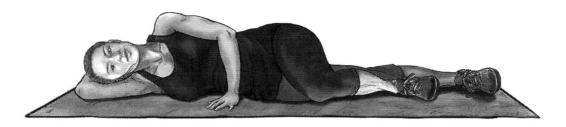

Begin exercising by slowly lifting your top leg one to three feet off the floor and holding for three seconds before slowly bringing your leg back to the starting position.

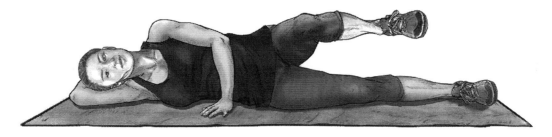

Perform 12 to 20 repetitions, then repeat on the opposite side.

Variations to Challenge Yourself

Single Leg Tuck with Weights: Follow the same instructions for the single leg tuck, except add ankle weights around the ankle of your top leg. Start with one or two pounds, and gradually increase the resistance.

Hip Adductor Squeeze

The hip adductor squeeze is performed on your back while squeezing a yoga block, bolster, or pillow that's three to five inches thick between your knees. This exercise targets your hip adductor muscles located on your inner thigh.

If you have groin or pubic bone issues, be careful with this exercise. Stop this exercise if it causes or increases pain in your pelvis, groin, or hips.

Step-by-Step Instructions

1. Get into the starting position:

   - Lie on your back with your knees bent and your feet flat on the floor.

   - Rest your arms next to your body with your palms flat on the floor and find pelvic neutral.

   - Place a yoga block, bolster, or pillow that's three to five inches thick between your knees, and squeeze as firmly as you can.

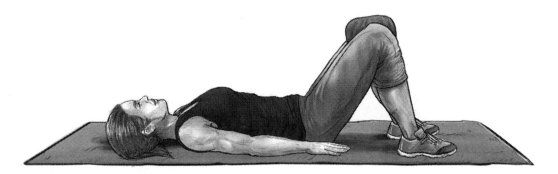

2. Brace your core by firing your pelvic floor and abdominal muscles while breathing to your belly button.

3. Begin exercising by slowly sliding your feet along the floor to extend your legs until your knees are straight. Pause for a second at the end of the motion, then slowly return your legs to the starting position. Be sure to maintain a firm squeeze on the yoga block, bolster, or pillow throughout this exercise.

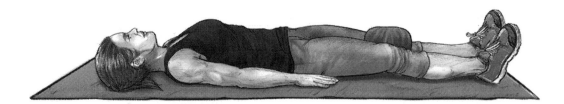

4. Perform 12 to 20 repetitions.

Common Mistakes

- **Using a bolster or pillow that's too thin:** If you're using a softer bolster or pillow for this exercise, it may be less than three inches thick once you squeeze it firmly between your knees, causing hip discomfort. Try folding the pillow or bolster in half or use more than one to ensure that it's three to five inches thick with a firm squeeze.

- **Not maintaining the firm squeeze:** Maintaining a firm squeeze throughout this exercise is important for effectively working your hip adductors. If you're unable to maintain a firm squeeze throughout this exercise, you may need to start with a modification for beginners.

- **Moving too fast:** Slowing it down will make this exercise more effective. Strive for a pace of three to five seconds to bring your legs forward and three to five seconds to return the legs to the starting position.

Modifications for Beginners

Static Hip Adductor Squeeze: Follow the same instructions for the hip adductor squeeze, except without moving your legs. Start with your knees bent and your feet flat on the floor. Begin exercising by squeezing the yoga block, bolster, or pillow as firmly as you can for three seconds, then lightly squeezing for three seconds. Alternate between firmly squeezing for three seconds and lightly squeezing for three seconds. Perform 12 to 20 repetitions.

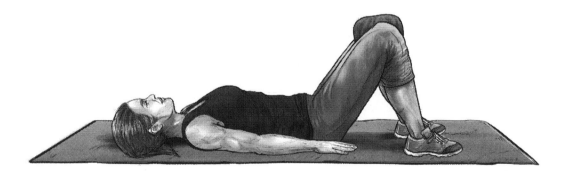

Variations to Challenge Yourself

Hip Adductor Squeeze with Legs Lifted: Follow the same instructions for the hip adductor squeeze, except keep your feet off the floor for this variation.

1. Start with your lower back pressed into the floor with your hips and your knees bent 90-degrees while firmly squeezing the yoga block, bolster, or pillow.

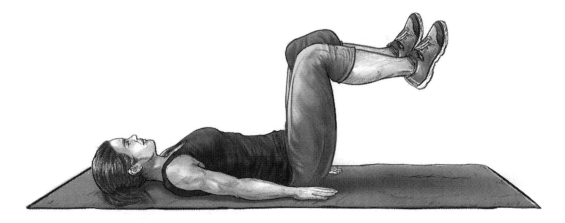

2. Begin exercising by slowly straightening and lowering both legs until the knees are straight and your feet are one to two feet above the floor. Pause for a second at the end of the motion, then slowly return your legs to the starting position. Be sure to maintain a firm squeeze on the yoga block, bolster, or pillow throughout this exercise.

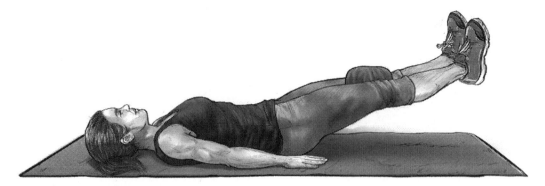

3. Perform 12 to 20 repetitions.

Hip Adductor Plank

The hip adductor plank, which is performed on your side, targets your hip adductor muscles located on your inner thigh. You'll need a chair, bench, or stool that's about one to two feet high for this exercise.

If you have groin or pubic bone issues, be careful with this exercise. Stop this exercise if it causes or increases pain in your pelvis, groin, or hips.

Step-by-Step Instructions

1. Get into the starting position:

    -   Lie on one side of your body with the inner side of your top foot on the chair, bench, or stool.

    -   Place your bottom elbow on the floor directly under your shoulder.

    -   Place your top hand on the top of your waist.

2. Brace your core by firing your pelvic floor and abdominal muscles while breathing to your belly button.

3. Begin exercising by lifting your torso off the floor so your body forms a straight line. Keep your knees hip-width apart with your bottom knee bent 90 degrees.

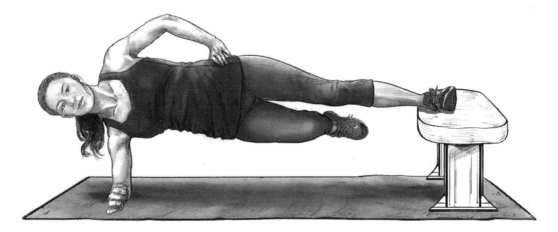

4. Hold for 30 to 60 seconds, then repeat on the opposite side.

Common Mistakes

- **Sagging your hips:** Your body should remain in a straight line between your knees and shoulders while your body is lifted. If you have difficulty keeping your hips from sagging, you may need to start with a modification for beginners.

- **Rotating your body:** If your body is rotated forward or backward during this exercise, it'll prevent you from working the correct muscles on your inner thigh. So make sure that your shoulders, hips, and legs are stacked on top of each other throughout this exercise. If you're unable to do this, you may need to start with a modification for beginners.

Modifications for Beginners

Bent-Knee Hip Adductor Plank on Chair: Follow the same instructions for the hip adductor plank, except with your top knee bent 90 degrees and the inner side of your top knee on the chair, bench, or stool.

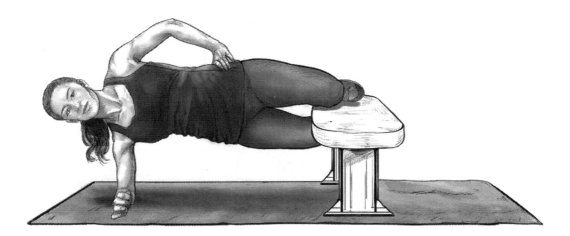

Variations to Challenge Yourself

Hip Adductor Plank with Weights: Follow the same instructions for the hip adductor plank, except place a dumbbell on your top waist and hold it in place with your top hand. Start with one pound, and gradually increase the resistance.

Hip Adductor Plank on Floor: Follow the same instructions for the hip adductor plank, except with the inner side of your top foot on the floor.

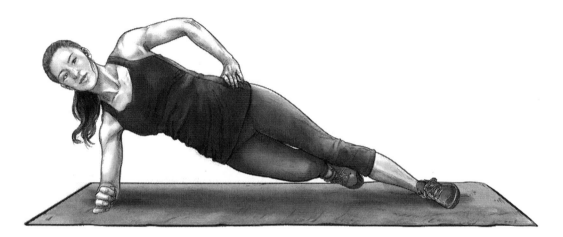

13. Stretching Exercises

Stretching is important for improving muscle flexibility and joint range of motion. By itself, stretching can help improve posture, relieve pain, and improve physical performance. Combining core and stretching exercises is a powerful way to help you quickly reach your goals.

Back and Hip Stretches

Single Leg Over Stretch

This stretch is performed on your back and targets your back and hip muscles.

Avoid this stretch if you have a history of spine surgery. Stop this stretch if it causes or increases pain in your back or hips.

Step-by-Step Instructions

1. Get into the starting position:

   - Lie on your back with one leg bent 90 degrees at the hip and knee.

   - Spread your arms to the sides of your body at about shoulder height.

   - Place your palms flat on the floor.

2. Take the hand on the opposite side of your bent leg and place it on top of the bent knee.

3. Pull your knee straight across your body toward the opposite hip while keeping the shoulders on the floor until you feel a good stretch in your hip or back.

4. Hold for 30 to 60 seconds, then repeat on the opposite side.

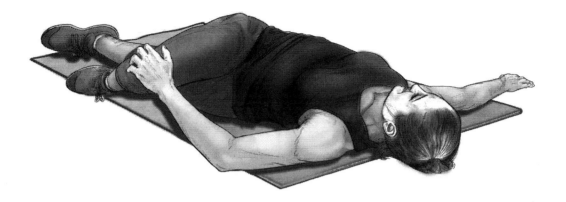

Common Mistakes

- **Letting your shoulders lift off the floor:** Make sure your shoulders stay glued to the floor to get the best results from this stretch.

- **Pulling your knee toward your chest:** You want to make sure to pull your bent knee straight across your body toward the opposite hip to get the best results from this stretch.

Seated Piriformis Stretch

This stretch is performed while sitting in a chair and targets your piriformis muscle in the buttocks.

Stop this stretch if it causes or increases pain in your knees or hips.

Step-by-Step Instructions

1. Get into the starting position:

   - Sit in a chair and cross the ankle of one leg over the knee of your other leg.

   - Place one hand on the ankle and the other hand on the knee of the crossed leg.

2. While keeping your spine straight, bend forward at the waist to bring your chest forward

until you feel a good stretch in your buttocks.

3.   Hold for 30 to 60 seconds, then repeat on the opposite side.

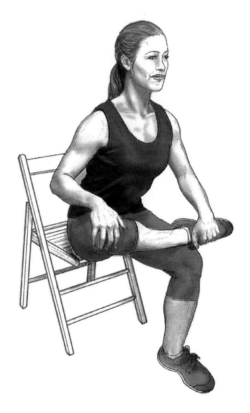

Common Mistakes

- **Rounding your spine:** Make sure your spine stays straight and that you're bending forward at the waist to get the best results from this stretch.

- **Letting your knee lift up:** If you let the knee of your crossed leg lift up, you won't get the full benefit, so make sure your knee stays about level with the ankle of the same leg. You can use your hand to push your knee down if needed.

Leg Stretches

Hamstring Towel Stretch

This stretch, which is performed on your back, targets your hamstring muscles on the back of your thigh. You'll need a belt or large towel for this stretch.

Stop this stretch if it causes or increases pain in your back, hips, or buttocks.

Step-by-Step Instructions

1. Get into the starting position:

   - Lie on your back with your knees bent and your feet on the floor.

   - Wrap a belt or center of a rolled-up towel around the ball of one foot while holding each end of the belt or towel in each hand.

2. Begin stretching by lifting and straightening your leg while pulling on the towel until you feel a good pull in the back of your thigh.

3. Hold for 30 to 60 seconds, then repeat on the opposite side.

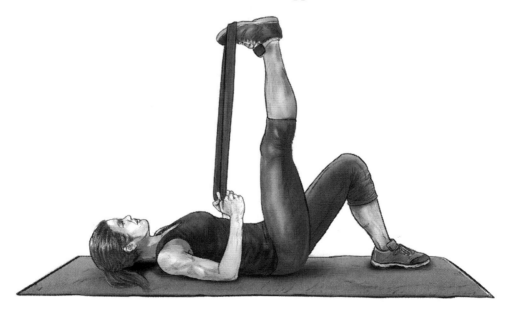

Common Mistakes

- **Bending your knee:** Bending your knee will make this stretch less effective, so make sure your knee stays straight by tightening your front thigh muscles (quadriceps).

- **Letting the leg drop to the side:** Make sure your leg is in line with your torso to get the best results from this stretch.

Side-Lying Quad Stretch

This stretch is performed while lying on your side and targets your quadriceps muscles on the front of your thigh. You may need a belt or towel for this stretch.

Stop this stretch if it causes or increases pain in your knees, hips, or back.

Step-by-Step Instructions

1. Get into the starting position:
   - Lie on one side of your body with your torso and legs in a straight line.
   - Rest your head on your bottom arm.
   - Bend your top leg and grasp your ankle with your top hand.

3. Begin stretching by gently thrusting your hips forward while pulling your heel toward your butt until you feel a good pull in the front of your thigh.

4. Hold for 30 to 60 seconds, then repeat on the opposite side.

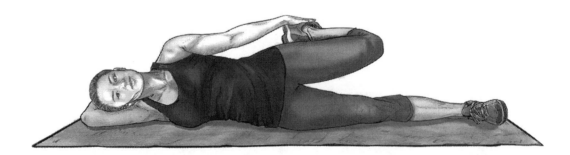

Common Mistakes

- **Bending your hips:** Since bending your hips will make this stretch less effective, make sure you're gently thrusting your hips forward so your body is in a straight line from your shoulders to your knees.

- **Lifting your knee too high:** You want to make sure your top knee is about hip-width apart from your bottom knee to get the best results from this stretch.

Modifications for Beginners

Quad Towel Stretch: If you have difficulty reaching your ankle, try wrapping a belt or the center of a rolled-up towel around your ankle and hold both ends of the belt or towel in your top hand.

Standing Calf Stretch

This stretch is performed while standing in front of a wall and targets your calf muscles on the back of your lower leg.

Stop this stretch if it causes or increases pain in your knees, ankles, or legs.

Step-by-Step Instructions

1. Get into the starting position:
   - Stand a few feet in front of a wall with your hands on the wall.
   - Take a big step back with the leg you want to stretch.
   - Make sure your back heel remains on the floor with your knee straight and toes pointed straight forward.

2. Begin stretching by bringing your hips forward until you feel a good pull on the back of your lower leg.

3. Hold for 30 to 60 seconds, then repeat on the opposite side.

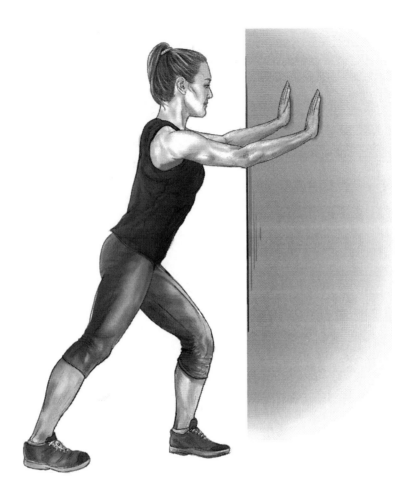

Common Mistakes

- **Bending your back knee:** Make sure your back knee is straight to get the best results from this stretch.

- **Lifting your back heel:** This stretch is less effective if your back heel is lifted off the floor, so keep your back heel pressed firmly to the floor.

- **Toes not pointing forward:** Keep your toes pointed straight forward to get the best results from this stretch.

Shoulder Stretches

Upper Trap Stretch

This stretch is performed while sitting in a chair and targets your upper trapezius muscle on the top of your shoulders.

Stop this stretch if it causes or increases pain in your neck or shoulders.

Step-by-Step Instructions

1. Get into the starting position:

    - Sit in a chair with your torso and head upright.

    - Hook one hand on the side of the seat and your other hand above your opposite ear.

2. Begin stretching by dropping your shoulders and gently pulling your head to the side until you feel a good pull in your upper trapezius muscle.

3. Hold for 30 to 60 seconds, then repeat on the opposite side.

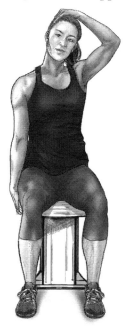

Common Mistakes

- **Dropping your head forward:** Make sure your head stays back so that your ears line up with your shoulders to get the best results from this stretch.

- **Shrugging your shoulders up:** If you shrug or lift your shoulders, you won't get the full benefit of this stretch. So make sure your shoulders stay down. Use the hand that's hooked on the side of the seat to help if needed.

Kneeling Lat Stretch

This stretch is performed on your knees with your arms on a chair and targets your latissimus dorsi muscle on the back of your torso.

Stop this stretch if it causes or increases pain in your back or shoulders.

Step-by-Step Instructions

1. Get into the starting position:

   - Kneel in front of a chair with your elbows shoulder-width apart on the seat of the chair and your knees hip-width apart directly under your hips.

   - Bend your elbows 90 degrees.

   - Keep your palms together and your fingers pointing toward the ceiling.

   - Place your head between your arms and aligned with your torso.

2. While keeping your spine straight and your elbows in place, begin stretching by tucking your tailbone under your body and slowly sitting your butt back toward your feet until you feel a good pull in your mid and upper back.

3. Hold for 30 to 60 seconds.

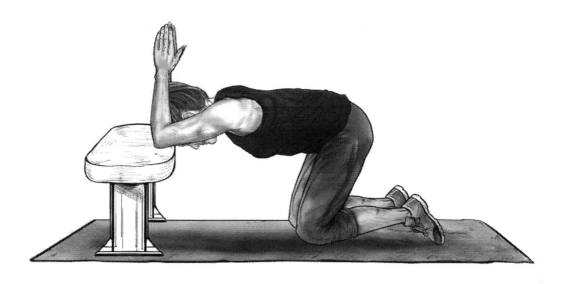

Common Mistakes

- **Arching your back:** To get the best results from this stretch, keep your spine straight or slightly rounded and tuck your tailbone under your body like you're thrusting your pelvis forward.

- **Palms not together:** Make sure your palms are together with your elbows bent 90 degrees to get the best results from this stretch.

Modifications for Beginners

Standing Lat Stretch: If you have difficulty getting on your knees, try performing this stretch while standing in front of a table or kitchen counter.

Wall Chest Stretch

This stretch is performed with one arm against a wall and targets your chest (pectoralis) and front of shoulder (anterior deltoid) muscles.

Avoid this stretch if you have a loose shoulder joint or if your shoulder dislocates. Stop this stretch if it causes or increases pain in your shoulders.

Step-by-Step Instructions

1. Get into the starting position:

   - Stand next to a wall.

   - Place your arm out to your side, with your elbow straight.

   - Place your fingers against the wall at about shoulder height.

2. Begin stretching by relaxing your shoulders down and rotating your body away from the hand that's on the wall until you feel a good pull in your chest.

3. Hold for 30 to 60 seconds, then repeat on the opposite side.

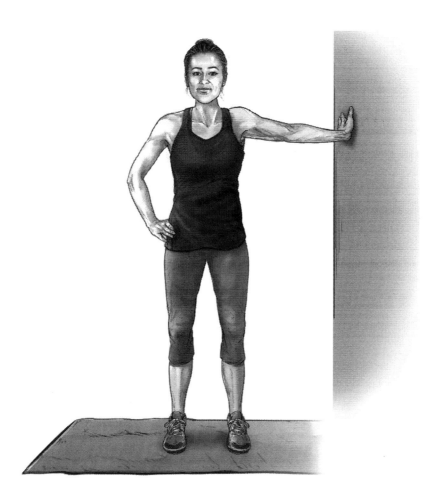

Common Mistakes

- **Bending your elbow:** If you bend your elbow while doing this stretch, you can put stress on your shoulder joint. So make sure to protect your shoulder by keeping your elbow straight.

- **Shrugging your shoulder up:** This stretch is less effective if you shrug or lift your shoulder. So make sure your shoulder stays down to get the best results from this stretch.

PART 4:

Core Workouts

Part 4 provides core workouts, consisting of four to five exercises, that are suitable for all ages, fitness levels, and goals.

Each chapter focuses on a different goal:

- chapter 14 — provides beginner to advanced workouts to develop a solid foundation of core strength to improve how you move and feel no matter who you are
- chapter 15 — improves posture
- chapter 16 — resolves back or knee pain
- chapter 17 — builds balance and prevent falls
- chapter 18 — prevents walking or running injuries to enhance performance

14. Beginner to Advanced Core Workouts

This chapter provides beginner, intermediate, and advanced core workouts for building a solid foundation of core strength so you can improve the way you move and feel. It doesn't matter if you're an older adult wanting to stay active, a new mom looking to rebuild your core after a recent pregnancy, or an athletic person seeking a performance edge. You'll see quick results by following the workouts below.

Begin by selecting a weekly program that fits your desired exercise time commitment, then select the workout that is appropriate for your fitness level.

Weekly Programs

Workouts that are longer than six minutes can be completed in one long session for a higher-intensity workout or split into six-minute sessions at different times during the day for a lower-intensity workout if you're in a pinch for time. Note: "x 2" or "x 3" means to perform the workout two or three times in a row, respectively.

6 Minutes, 2 x a Week

- Day 1: Torso workout
- Day 3, 4, or 5: Torso workout

6 Minutes, 3 x a Week

- Day 1: Torso workout
- Day 3: Torso workout
- Day 5: Torso workout

or

- Day 1: Torso workout
- Day 3: Hip or shoulder workout

- Day 5: Torso workout

or

- Day 1: Torso workout
- Day 3: Hip workout
- Day 5: Shoulder workout

6 Minutes, 4 x a Week

- Day 1: Torso workout
- Day 2: Hip workout
- Day 3: Torso workout
- Day 4: Shoulder workout

6 Minutes, 5 x a Week

- Day 1: Torso workout
- Day 2: Hip workout
- Day 3: Torso workout
- Day 4: Shoulder workout
- Day 5: Torso workout

12 Minutes, 2 x a Week

- Day 1: Torso workout x 2
- Day 3, 4, or 5: Torso workout x 2

or

- Day 1: Torso workout, hip workout
- Day 3, 4, or 5: Torso workout, shoulder workout

12 Minutes, 3 x a Week

- Day 1: Torso workout x 2
- Day 3: Hip workout, shoulder workout
- Day 5: Torso workout x 2

or

- Day 1: Torso workout, hip workout
- Day 3: Torso workout, shoulder workout
- Day 5: Torso workout, hip or shoulder workout

or

- Day 1: Torso workout x 2
- Day 3: Hip workout x 2
- Day 5: Shoulder workout x 2

12 Minutes, 4 x a Week

- Day 1: Torso workout x 2
- Day 2: Hip workout x 2
- Day 3: Torso workout x 2
- Day 4: Shoulder workout x 2

12 Minutes, 5 x a Week

- Day 1: Torso workout x 2
- Day 2: Hip workout x 2
- Day 3: Torso workout x 2
- Day 4: Shoulder workout x 2
- Day 5: Torso workout x 2

18 Minutes, 2 x a Week

- Day 1: Torso workout x 2, hip workout

- Day 3, 4, or 5: Torso workout x 2, shoulder workout

or

- Day 1: Torso workout, hip workout, shoulder workout

- Day 3, 4, or 5: Torso workout, hip workout, shoulder workout

18 Minutes, 3 x a Week

- Day 1: Torso workout x 2, hip workout

- Day 3: Torso workout x 2, shoulder workout

- Day 5: Torso workout x 2, hip or shoulder workout

or

- Day 1: Torso workout x 3

- Day 3: Hip workout x 3

- Day 5: Shoulder workout x 3

or

- Day 1: Torso workout, hip workout, shoulder workout

- Day 3: Torso workout, hip workout, shoulder workout

- Day 5: Torso workout, hip workout, shoulder workout

Workouts

Complete each exercise in the order suggested, with little to no rest between exercises. Skip exercises that don't work for you, and substitute ones that are too easy or too difficult. If you find the exercises too easy, move on to the next level. Review the exercise instructions in part 3 as needed.

Beginner Workouts

If you're new to core exercises, getting back into exercise after a long break, or recovering from an injury, use these workouts.

TORSO WORKOUT

1. Dead bug ——————————

2. Bird dog ——————————

3. Side plank on knees ——————————

4. Static leg lift with knees bent ——————————

5. Anti-rotation wall press ——————————

HIP WORKOUT

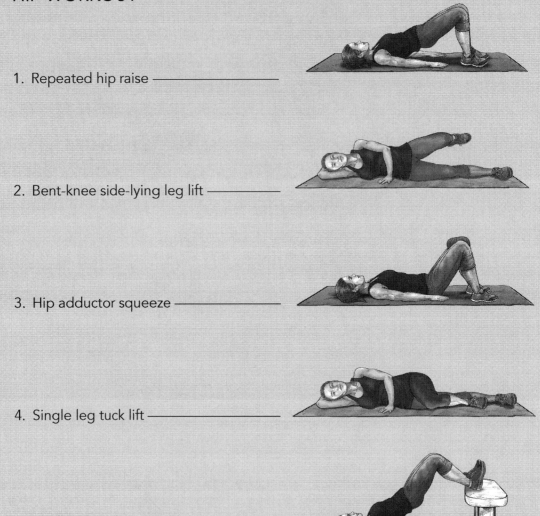

1. Repeated hip raise ————————————

2. Bent-knee side-lying leg lift ————————

3. Hip adductor squeeze ——————————

4. Single leg tuck lift ——————————

5. Double leg heel bridge ————————

SHOULDER WORKOUT

1. T arm lift ————————————————————

2. U arm lift ————————————————————

3. Y arm lift ————————————————————

4. Wall push ————————————————————

Intermediate Workouts

The intermediate workouts are appropriate if you have some experience with core exercises and are in decent shape.

TORSO WORKOUT

1. Front plank ————————————

2. Bird dog with weights ————————————

3. Side plank ————————————

4. Static leg lift ————————————

5. Oblique half twist ————————————

HIP WORKOUT

1. Hip raise ———————————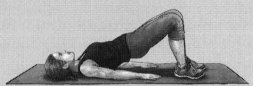

2. Side-lying leg lift ————————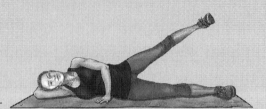

3. Hip adductor squeeze with legs lifted —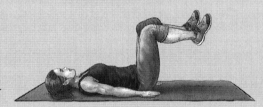

4. Single leg tuck ———————————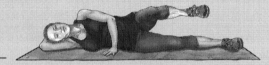

5. Heel bridge with marches ———————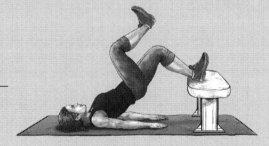

SHOULDER WORKOUT

1. T arm lift with weights ————————

2. U arm lift with weights ————————

3. Y arm lift with weights ————————

4. Floor push ————————

Advanced Workouts

If you have a lot of experience with core exercises and are in great shape, you are ready for the advanced workouts.

TORSO WORKOUT

1. Static leg lifts with weights

2. Modified superman with weights

3. Side body lift with weights

4. Static trunk lift with weights

5. Resistance band anti-rotation press

HIP WORKOUT

1. Single leg hip raise ————————

2. Side-lying leg lift with weights ————

3. Hip adductor plank ——————————

4. Single leg tuck with weights ————

5. Single leg heel bridge ——————————

SHOULDER WORKOUT

1. T arm lift with weights ———————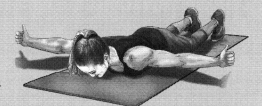

2. U arm lift with weights ———————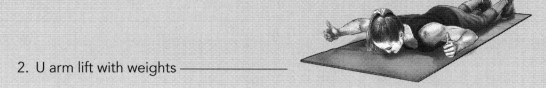

3. Y arm lift with weights ———————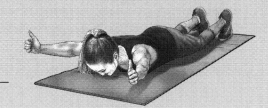

4. Floor push with weights ———————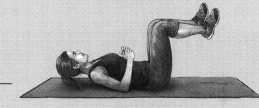

5. TUY arm lift with weights ————————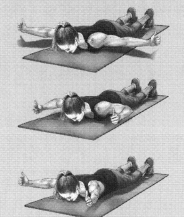

15. Improve Posture

With poor posture, you sit or stand with your head forward, shoulders rounded, and back slouched, which can lead to pain or discomfort in the neck, shoulders, arms, and back. Additionally, movement becomes more cumbersome because the body is out of alignment.

With good posture, you sit or stand upright with your head on top of your shoulders and your shoulders on top of your hips. Good posture will help you move with less pain and more ease. It'll also boost your confidence and positively impact the way people perceive you.

Luckily, posture is easier to address than most people realize, and you can improve your posture even if it's been a problem for years. Follow these simple workouts that combine core strengthening and stretching exercises to develop good posture so you can stand upright and move with more grace, confidence, and ease.

Perform the posture workouts for the weekly program that fits your exercise time commitment.

Weekly Programs

Workouts that are longer than six minutes can be completed in one long session for a higher-intensity workout or split into six-minute sessions at different times during the day for a lower-intensity workout if you're in a pinch for time. Note: "x 2" or "x 3" means to perform the workout two or three times in a row, respectively.

6 Minutes, 2 x a Week

- Day 1: Posture workout A
- Day 3, 4, or 5: Posture workout B

6 Minutes, 3 x a Week

- Day 1: Posture workout A
- Day 3: Posture workout B
- Day 5: Posture workout A or B

6 Minutes, 4 x a Week

- Day 1: Posture workout C
- Day 2: Posture workout D
- Day 3: Posture workout C
- Day 4: Posture workout D

6 Minutes, 5 x a Week

- Day 1: Posture workout C
- Day 2: Posture workout D
- Day 3: Posture workout C
- Day 4: Posture workout D
- Day 5: Posture workout C

12 Minutes, 2 x a Week

- Day 1: Posture workout C x 2
- Day 3, 4, or 5: Posture workout D x 2

12 Minutes, 3 x a Week

- Day 1: Posture workout C x 2
- Day 3: Posture workout D x 2
- Day 5: Posture workout C x 2

12 Minutes, 4 x a Week

- Day 1: Posture workout C x 2
- Day 2: Posture workout D x 2
- Day 3: Posture workout C x 2
- Day 4: Posture workout D x 2

12 Minutes, 5 x a Week

- Day 1: Posture workout C x 2
- Day 2: Posture workout D x 2
- Day 3: Posture workout C x 2
- Day 4: Posture workout D x 2
- Day 5: Posture workout C x 2

18 Minutes, 2 x a Week

- Day 1: Posture workout C x 3
- Day 3, 4, or 5: Posture workout D x 3

18 Minutes, 3 x a Week

- Day 1: Posture workout C x 3
- Day 3: Posture workout D x 3
- Day 5: Posture workout C x 3

Posture Workouts

Complete each exercise in the order suggested, with little to no rest between exercises. Skip the exercises that don't work for you, and substitute ones that are too easy or too difficult. Review the exercise instructions in part 3 as needed.

POSTURE WORKOUT A

1. Hip raise ————————————————

2. Side plank ————————————————

3. TUY arm lift ————————————————

4. Side-lying quad stretch ——————————

5. Kneeling lat stretch ——————————

POSTURE WORKOUT B

1. Front plank ————————————

2. Floor press ————————————

3. Bird dog ——————————————

4. Wall chest stretch ——————————

5. Upper trap stretch ——————————

POSTURE WORKOUT C

1. Hip raise ——————————

2. Front plank ——————————

3. TUY arm lift ——————————

4. Floor press ——————————

5. Bird dog ——————————

POSTURE WORKOUT D

1. Side-lying quad stretch —————————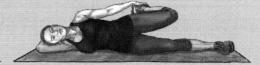

2. Kneeling lat stretch —————————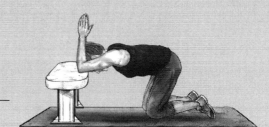

3. Wall chest stretch —————————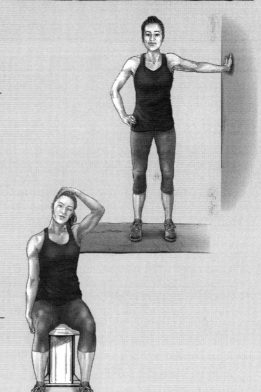

4. Upper trap stretch —————————

16. Relieve Back and Knee Pain

People most commonly experience pain in their back and knees. By using these workouts that combine core strengthening and stretching exercises, you can relieve your back and knee pain.

Whether you have upper back pain or lower back pain, your pain can be a result of weak abdominal and hip muscles that forces the back muscles to work harder. Research shows strengthening core muscles is effective for relieving back pain.[20] Pain can also be a result of tight muscles, such as the hamstrings or latissimus dorsi, and stretching these muscles may reduce back pain. Additional ways to steer clear of back pain include maintaining good posture and using the proper lifting technique. To maintain good posture, sit or stand upright with your head on top of your shoulders and your shoulders on top of your hips. (See chapter 15 for workouts to improve posture.) The proper technique is to use your legs instead of your back when lifting. Do this by bending at the hips and knees while keeping your back straight and core braced when lifting something heavy.

Knee pain is typically located at the front of the knee or around the kneecap because of squatting, stair climbing, walking, running, or jumping. Research shows that strengthening the hips and abdominal muscles is effective for relieving knee pain.[21] Tight hamstring and quadricep muscles are also common contributors to pain and stretching these muscles may also reduce knee pain.[22]

Perform the back or knee workouts for the weekly program that fits your exercise time commitment.

Weekly Programs

Workouts that are longer than six minutes can be completed in one long session for a higher-intensity workout or split into six-minute sessions at different times during the day for a lower-intensity workout if you're in a pinch for time. Note: "x 2" or "x 3" means to perform the workout two or three times in a row, respectively.

6 Minutes, 2 x a Week

- Day 1: Back/Knee workout A

- Day 3, 4, or 5: Back/Knee workout B

6 Minutes, 3 x a Week

- Day 1: Back/Knee workout A

- Day 3: Back/Knee workout B

- Day 5: Back/Knee workout A or B

6 Minutes, 4 x a Week

- Day 1: Back/Knee workout C

- Day 2: Back/Knee workout D

- Day 3: Back/Knee workout C

- Day 4: Back/Knee workout D

6 Minutes, 5 x a Week

- Day 1: Back/Knee workout C

- Day 2: Back/Knee workout D

- Day 3: Back/Knee workout C

- Day 4: Back/Knee workout D

- Day 5: Back/Knee workout C

12 Minutes, 2 x a Week

- Day 1: Back/Knee workout C x 2

- Day 3, 4, or 5: Back/Knee workout D x 2

12 Minutes, 3 x a Week

- Day 1: Back/Knee workout C x 2
- Day 3: Back/Knee workout D x 2
- Day 5: Back/Knee workout C x 2

12 Minutes, 4 x a Week

- Day 1: Back/Knee workout C x 2
- Day 2: Back/Knee workout D x 2
- Day 3: Back/Knee workout C x 2
- Day 4: Back/Knee workout D x 2

12 Minutes, 5 x a Week

- Day 1: Back/Knee workout C x 2
- Day 2: Back/Knee workout D x 2
- Day 3: Back/Knee workout C x 2
- Day 4: Back/Knee workout D x 2
- Day 5: Back/Knee workout C x 2

18 Minutes, 2 x a Week

- Day 1: Back/Knee workout C x 3
- Day 3, 4, or 5: Back/Knee workout D x 3

18 Minutes, 3 x a Week

- Day 1: Back/Knee workout C x 3
- Day 3: Back/Knee workout D x 3
- Day 5: Back/Knee workout C x 3

Back Workouts

Complete each exercise in the order suggested, with little to no rest between exercises. Skip the exercises that don't work for you, and substitute ones that are too easy or too difficult. Review the exercise instructions in part 3 as needed.

BACK WORKOUT A

1. Bird dog —————————————

2. Side plank —————————————

3. Dead bug —————————————

4. Single leg over stretch —————————

5. Hamstring towel stretch —————————

BACK WORKOUT B

1. Static leg lift ────────────────

2. Side-lying leg lift ──────────────

3. Hip adductor squeeze ────────────

4. Seated piriformis stretch ──────────

5. Kneeling lat stretch ────────────

BACK WORKOUT C

1. Bird dog ————————————————

2. Side plank ————————————————

3. Static leg lift ————————————————

4. Side-lying leg lift ————————————————

5. Hip adductor squeeze ————————————————

BACK WORKOUT D

1. Single leg over stretch ————————

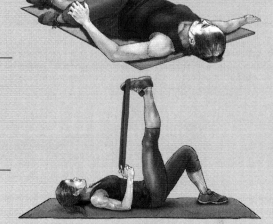

2. Hamstring towel stretch ————————

3. Seated piriformis stretch ————————

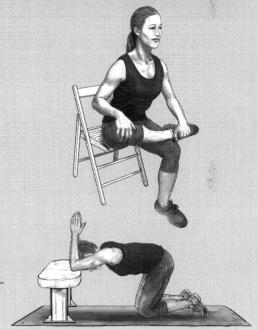

4. Kneeling lat stretch ————————

Knee Workouts

KNEE WORKOUT A

1. Side-lying leg lift ————————————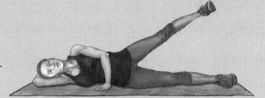

2. Hip raise —————————————————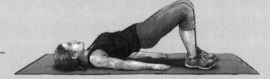

3. Hip adductor squeeze —————————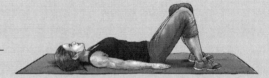

4. Single leg over stretch ————————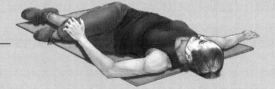

5. Side-lying quad stretch —————————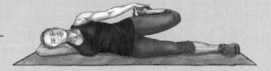

KNEE WORKOUT B

1. Heel bridge with marches ———————

2. Single leg tuck ———————————

3. Front plank ——————————————

4. Side body lift ——————————————

5. Hamstring towel stretch ————————

KNEE WORKOUT C

1. Side-lying leg lift ————————————

2. Hip raise ————————————

3. Hip adductor squeeze ————————————

4. Heel bridge with marches ————————————

5. Single leg tuck ————————————

KNEE WORKOUT D

1. Front plank ————————————

2. Side body lift ————————————

3. Single leg over stretch ——————

4. Hamstring towel stretch ————————

5. Side-lying quad stretch ——————————

17. Build Balance and Prevent Falls

Core exercises train the muscles of your abdominals, back, and hips to work in harmony. This leads to better balance and stability, which reduces the risk of falling and improves the ease of performing daily activities, such as getting up from a chair, walking, or climbing stairs. Interestingly, research has shown that core exercises are more effective than traditional balance and strength exercises for improving balance and preventing falls in older adults.[23] Most higher-intensity physical activities, like those involved in traditional fitness routines and sports, also depend on strong core muscles to keep your body upright and balanced.

Perform the balance workouts for the weekly program that fits your exercise time commitment.

Weekly Programs

Workouts that are longer than six minutes can be completed in one long session for a higher-intensity workout or split into six-minute sessions at different times during the day for a lower-intensity workout if you're in a pinch for time. Note: "x 2" or "x 3" means to perform the workout two or three times in a row, respectively.

6 Minutes, 2 x a Week

- Day 1: Balance workout A
- Day 3, 4, or 5: Balance workout B

6 Minutes, 3 x a Week

- Day 1: Balance workout A
- Day 3: Balance workout B
- Day 5: Balance workout A or B

6 Minutes, 4 x a Week

- Day 1: Balance workout C
- Day 2: Balance workout D
- Day 3: Balance workout C
- Day 4: Balance workout D

6 Minutes, 5 x a Week

- Day 1: Balance workout C
- Day 2: Balance workout D
- Day 3: Balance workout C
- Day 4: Balance workout D
- Day 5: Balance workout C

12 Minutes, 2 x a Week

- Day 1: Balance workout C x 2
- Day 3, 4, or 5: Balance workout D x 2

12 Minutes, 3 x a Week

- Day 1: Balance workout C x 2
- Day 3: Balance workout D x 2
- Day 5: Balance workout C x 2

12 Minutes, 4 x a Week

- Day 1: Balance workout C x 2
- Day 2: Balance workout D x 2

- Day 3: Balance workout C x 2
- Day 4: Balance workout D x 2

12 Minutes, 5 x a Week

- Day 1: Balance workout C x 2
- Day 2: Balance workout D x 2
- Day 3: Balance workout C x 2
- Day 4: Balance workout D x 2
- Day 5: Balance workout C x 2

18 Minutes, 2 x a Week

- Day 1: Balance workout C x 3
- Day 3, 4, or 5: Balance workout D x 3

18 Minutes, 3 x a Week

- Day 1: Balance workout C x 3
- Day 3: Balance workout D x 3
- Day 5: Balance workout C x 3

Balance Workouts

Complete each exercise in the order suggested, with little to no rest between exercises. Skip the exercises that don't work for you, and substitute ones that are too easy or too difficult. Review the exercise instructions in part 3 as needed.

BALANCE WORKOUT A

1. Front plank ————————————

2. Side plank ————————————

3. Bird dog ————————————

4. Side-lying leg lift ————————————

5. Single leg stance ————————————

BALANCE WORKOUT B

1. Static leg lift —————————

2. Anti-rotation wall press —————

3. Hip raise ——————————————

4. Hip adductor squeeze ——————

5. Single leg stance ————————

BALANCE WORKOUT C

1. Front plank —————————————————

2. Bird dog —————————————————

3. Static leg lift —————————————————

4. Hip raise —————————————————

5. Single leg stance —————————————————

BALANCE WORKOUT D

1. Anti-rotation wall press ────────────

2. Side-lying leg lift ────────────────

3. Side plank ──────────────────────

4. Hip adductor squeeze ──────────────

5. Single leg stance ─────────────────

18. Prevent Walking or Running Injuries and Enhance Performance

Walking and running are the most popular forms of exercise worldwide. In the United States, half of the population use walking or running for exercise as part of a physically active lifestyle. This makes sense because walking and running are great ways to get in shape, relieve stress, and have fun. It's also completely free because no special equipment or training is needed. However, you can experience back, hip, knee, or ankle pain because of walking or running. Luckily, core exercises combined with stretching can help prevent walking- and running-related pain and injuries while also enhancing performance.

Research shows that exercising core muscles before activities such as walking and running can immediately change the stiffness of the muscles, which can improve physical performance and injury resilience.[24] It's also well-known that stretching improves the flexibility of your muscles and the range of motion of your joints. And having better flexibility and range of motion enables your body to work more effectively, which also enhances physical performance and decreases the risk of injuries.

Perform the warmup exercises immediately before and the cooldown exercises immediately after walking or running to prevent injuries and improve performance. Perform them in the order suggested, with little to no rest in between the exercises. Skip the ones that don't work for you, and substitute ones that are too easy or difficult. Review the exercise instructions in part 3 as needed.

WARMUP

Perform each exercise before walking or running.

1. Front plank ————————

2. Side plank ————————

3. Heel bridge with marches ————

4. Single leg tuck ————————

5. Hip adductor squeeze ————————

COOLDOWN

Perform each stretch after walking or running.

1. Single leg over stretch ———————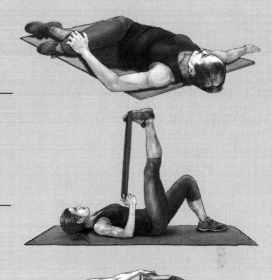

2. Hamstring towel stretch ———————

3. Side-lying quad stretch ———————

4. Seated piriformis stretch ———————

5. Standing calf stretch ———————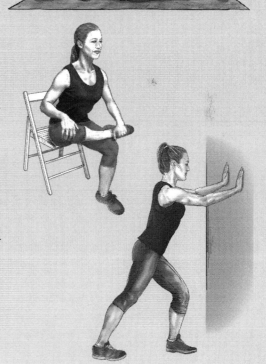

Conclusion

Congratulations on completing *6-Minute Core Strength*!

You're now empowered with the knowledge and skills to transform your body and your life, no matter your age, weight, or fitness level.

I hope you'll use what you've learned in this book to move, feel, and live better than you ever have before!

Would You Do Me a Favor?

I have a small favor to ask: Would you take a minute to write a review of this book on Amazon? I check all my reviews and would love to get your honest feedback. The true satisfaction I get from this work is knowing how I'm helping people.

To leave me a review:

- You can visit www.sixminutefitness.com/corereview, and you'll be automatically taken to Amazon to leave a review.

- You can also pull up Amazon on your web browser, search for "6-Minute Core Strength," click on the link for this book, scroll down, and click on "Write a customer review."

Thanks again, and I look forward to reading your feedback!

About the Author

Dr. Jonathan Su is a physical therapist and fitness expert whose mission is to make fitness accessible for everyone, no matter their age, weight, or fitness level. Dr. Su is coauthor of the clinical textbook *Netter's Orthopaedic Clinical Examination* and the bestselling author of *Six-Minute Fitness at 60+*.

Dr. Su is a former U.S. Army officer in charge of injury prevention, rehabilitation, and performance optimization for over 4,500 active-duty soldiers in the field. This experience helped him develop expertise in tactical fitness and rapid rehabilitation using little to no equipment.

When not busy writing or working with clients, you can find him exploring hole-in-the-wall restaurants and spending quality time outdoors with his family.

References

1. Granacher, Urs, Andre Lacroix, Thomas Muehlbauer, Katrin Roettger, and Albert Gollhofer. "Effects of Core Instability Strength Training on Trunk Muscle Strength, Spinal Mobility, Dynamic Balance and Functional Mobility in Older Adults." *Gerontology* 59, no. 2 (2013): 105–13. https://doi.org/10.1159/000343152. Kibler, W. Ben, Joel Press, and Aaron Sciascia. "The Role of Core Stability in Athletic Function." *Sports Medicine (Auckland, N.Z.)* 36, no. 3 (2006): 189–98. https://doi.org/10.2165/00007256-200636030-00001. Kim, Beomryong, and Jongeun Yim. "Core Stability and Hip Exercises Improve Physical Function and Activity in Patients with Non-Specific Low Back Pain: A Randomized Controlled Trial." *The Tohoku Journal of Experimental Medicine* 251, no. 3 (July 2020): 193–206. https://doi.org/10.1620/tjem.251.193.

2. Sharrock, Chris, Jarrod Cropper, Joel Mostad, Matt Johnson, and Terry Malone. "A PILOT STUDY OF CORE STABILITY AND ATHLETIC PERFORMANCE: IS THERE A RELATIONSHIP?" *International Journal of Sports Physical Therapy* 6, no. 2 (June 2011): 63–74. https://www.ncbi.nlm.nih.gov/pmc/articles/PMC3109894/.

3. Hibbs, Angela E., Kevin G. Thompson, Duncan French, Allan Wrigley, and Iain Spears. "Optimizing Performance by Improving Core Stability and Core Strength." *Sports Medicine (Auckland, N.Z.)* 38, no. 12 (2008): 995–1008. https://doi.org/10.2165/00007256-200838120-00004.

4. Callaghan, J. P., and S. M. McGill. "Low Back Joint Loading and Kinematics during Standing and Unsupported Sitting." *Ergonomics* 44, no. 3 (February 20, 2001): 280–94. https://doi.org/10.1080/00140130118276.

5. Shinkle, Justin, Thomas W. Nesser, Timothy J. Demchak, and David M. McMannus. "Effect of Core Strength on the Measure of Power in the Extremities." *Journal of Strength and Conditioning Research* 26, no. 2 (February 2012): 373–80. https://doi.org/10.1519/JSC.0b013e31822600e5.

6. Häggmark, T., and A. Thorstensson. "Fibre Types in Human Abdominal Muscles." *Acta Physiologica Scandinavica* 107, no. 4 (December 1979): 319–25. https://doi.org/10.1111/j.1748-1716.1979.tb06482.x. Thorstensson, A., and H. Carlson. "Fibre Types in Human Lumbar Back Muscles." *Acta Physiologica Scandinavica* 131, no. 2 (October 1987): 195–202. https://doi.org/10.1111/j.1748-1716.1987.tb08226.x.

7. Callaghan, J. P., and S. M. McGill. "Intervertebral Disc Herniation: Studies on a Porcine Model Exposed to Highly Repetitive Flexion/Extension Motion with Compressive Force." *Clinical Biomechanics (Bristol, Avon)* 16, no. 1 (January 2001): 28–37. https://doi.org/10.1016/s0268-0033(00)00063-2.

8. Tampier, Claudio, Janessa D. M. Drake, Jack P. Callaghan, and Stuart M. McGill. "Progressive Disc Herniation: An Investigation of the Mechanism Using Radiologic, Histochemical, and Microscopic Dissection Techniques on a Porcine Model." *Spine* 32, no. 25 (December 1, 2007): 2869–74. https://doi.org/10.1097/BRS.0b013e31815b64f5.

9. Thoreson, Olof, Lars Ekström, Hans-Arne Hansson, Carl Todd, Wisam Witwit, Anna Swärd Aminoff, Pall Jonasson, and Adad Baranto. "The Effect of Repetitive Flexion and Extension Fatigue Loading on the Young Porcine Lumbar Spine, a Feasibility Study of MRI and Histological Analyses." *Journal of Experimental Orthopaedics* 4, no. 1 (December 2017): 16. https://doi.org/10.1186/s40634-017-0091-7.

10. McGill, Stuart. "Core Training: Evidence Translating to Better Performance and Injury Prevention." *Strength & Conditioning Journal* 32, no. 3 (June 2010): 33–46. https://doi.org/10.1519/SSC.0b013e3181df4521.

11. Holm, S., and A. Nachemson. "Variations in the Nutrition of the Canine Intervertebral Disc Induced by Motion." *Spine* 8, no. 8 (December 1983): 866–74. https://doi.org/10.1097/00007632-198311000-00009.

12. Stevens, Sjoerd, Anouk Agten, Annick Timmermans, and Frank Vandenabeele. "Unilateral Changes of the Multifidus in Persons with Lumbar Disc Herniation: A Systematic Review and Meta-Analysis." *The Spine Journal: Official Journal of the North American Spine Society* 20, no. 10 (October 2020): 1573–85. https://doi.org/10.1016/j.spinee.2020.04.007.

13. Uber-Zak, Lori D., and Y. Swamy Venkatesh. "Neurologic Complications of Sit-Ups Associated with the Valsalva Maneuver: 2 Case Reports." *Archives of Physical Medicine and Rehabilitation* 83, no. 2 (February 2002): 278–82. https://doi.org/10.1053/apmr.2002.27378.

14. Childs, John D., Deydre S. Teyhen, Timothy M. Benedict, Jamie B. Morris, Andrew D. Fortenberry, Rene M. McQueen, Janice B. Preston, Alison C. Wright, Jessica L. Dugan, and Steven Z. George. "Effects of Sit-up Training versus Core Stabilization Exercises on Sit-up Performance." *Medicine and Science in Sports and Exercise* 41, no. 11 (November 2009): 2072–83. https://doi.org/10.1249/MSS.0b013e3181a84db2.

15. Macfarlane, Duncan J., Lynne H. Taylor, and Thomas F. Cuddihy. "Very Short Intermittent vs Continuous Bouts of Activity in Sedentary Adults." *Preventive Medicine* 43, no. 4 (October 2006): 332–36. https://doi.org/10.1016/j.ypmed.2006.06.002.

16. Jakicic, J. M., R. R. Wing, B. A. Butler, and R. J. Robertson. "Prescribing Exercise in Multiple Short Bouts versus One Continuous Bout: Effects on Adherence, Cardiorespiratory Fitness, and Weight Loss in Overweight Women." *International Journal of Obesity and Related Metabolic Disorders: Journal of the International Association for the Study of Obesity* 19, no. 12 (December 1995): 893–901.

17. Kelleher, Andrew R., Kyle J. Hackney, Timothy J. Fairchild, Stefan Keslacy, and Lori L. Ploutz-Snyder. "The Metabolic Costs of Reciprocal Supersets vs. Traditional Resistance Exercise in Young Recreationally Active Adults." *Journal of Strength and Conditioning Research* 24, no. 4 (April 2010): 1043–51. https://doi.org/10.1519/JSC.0b013e3181d3e993.

18. Realzola, Rogelio A., Zachary A. Mang, Desmond J. Millender, Jason R. Beam, Bryanne N. Bellovary, Andrew D. Wells, Jonathan M. Houck, and Len Kravitz. "Metabolic Profile of Reciprocal Supersets in Young, Recreationally Active Women and Men." *Journal of Strength and Conditioning Research*, April 27, 2021. https://doi.org/10.1519/JSC.0000000000003920.

19. Allison, Garry T., Sue L. Morris, and Brendan Lay. "Feedforward Responses of Transversus Abdominis Are Directionally Specific and Act Asymmetrically: Implications for Core Stability Theories." *The Journal of Orthopaedic and Sports Physical Therapy* 38, no. 5 (May 2008): 228–37. https://doi.org/10.2519/jospt.2008.2703.

20. Wang, Xue-Qiang, Jie-Jiao Zheng, Zhuo-Wei Yu, Xia Bi, Shu-Jie Lou, Jing Liu, Bin Cai, et al. "A Meta-Analysis of Core Stability Exercise versus General Exercise for Chronic Low Back Pain." *PloS One* 7, no. 12 (2012): e52082. https://doi.org/10.1371/journal.pone.0052082.

21. Ferber, Reed, Lori Bolgla, Jennifer E. Earl-Boehm, Carolyn Emery, and Karrie Hamstra-Wright. "Strengthening of the Hip and Core versus Knee Muscles for the Treatment of Patellofemoral Pain: A Multicenter Randomized Controlled Trial." *Journal of Athletic Training* 50, no. 4 (April 2015): 366–77. https://doi.org/10.4085/1062-6050-49.3.70.

22. Lee, Jin Hyuck, Ki-Mo Jang, Eunseon Kim, Hye Chang Rhim, and Hyeong-Dong Kim. "Effects of Static and Dynamic Stretching With Strengthening Exercises in Patients With Patellofemoral Pain Who Have Inflexible Hamstrings: A Randomized Controlled Trial." *Sports Health* 13, no. 1 (February 2021): 49–56. https://doi.org/10.1177/1941738120932911. Lee, Jin Hyuck, Ki-Mo Jang, Eunseon Kim, Hye Chang Rhim, and Hyeong-Dong Kim. "Static and Dynamic Quadriceps Stretching Exercises in Patients With Patellofemoral Pain: A Randomized Controlled Trial." *Sports Health* 13, no. 5 (October 2021): 482–89. https://doi.org/10.1177/1941738121993777.

23. Granacher, Urs, Albert Gollhofer, Tibor Hortobágyi, Reto W. Kressig, and Thomas Muehlbauer. "The Importance of Trunk Muscle Strength for Balance, Functional Performance, and Fall Prevention in Seniors: A Systematic Review." *Sports Medicine (Auckland, N.Z.)* 43, no. 7 (July 2013): 627–41. https://doi.org/10.1007/s40279-013-0041-1.

24. Lee, Benjamin, and Stuart McGill. "The Effect of Short-Term Isometric Training on Core/Torso Stiffness." *Journal of Sports Sciences* 35, no. 17 (September 2017): 1724–33. https://doi.org/10.1080/02640414.2016.1235791.

Free Bonus Material

I want to make sure you get as much value as possible from this book, so I've put together a few additional free bonus materials to help you, including:

- Videos demonstrating each exercise and their variations to increase or decrease the difficulty level

- Workout plans neatly laid out and provided in PDF and Excel formats

- A monthly email newsletter with tips to help you succeed on your health and fitness journey

To get instant access to all of this free bonus material, go here now:
www.sixminutefitness.com/corebonus

And if you have any questions or run into any difficulties, just shoot me an email at jonathan@sixminutefitness.com, and I'll do my best to help!

Made in the USA
Middletown, DE
15 April 2024

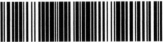